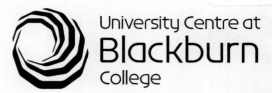

University Centre at
Blackburn
College

Telephone: 01254 292165

Please return this book on or before the last date shown

26th Sept 14.	
24th Oct 14.	

other titles in the series

PRINCIPLES OF

CHINESE HERBAL MEDICINE

What it is, how it works, and what it can do for you

Revised Edition

John Hicks

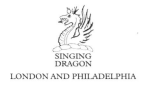

SINGING
DRAGON

LONDON AND PHILADELPHIA

This edition published in 2013
by Singing Dragon
an imprint of Jessica Kingsley Publishers
116 Pentonville Road
London N1 9JB, UK
and
400 Market Street, Suite 400
Philadelphia, PA 19106, USA

www.singingdragon.com

First published in 1997 by Thorsons, an imprint of HarperCollins

Library of Congress Cataloging in Publication Data
Hicks, John (Herbalist)
  [Thorsons principles of Chinese herbal medicine]
  Principles of Chinese herbal medicine / John Hicks.
      pages cm
  Revision of the author's: Thorsons principles of Chinese herbal medicine, 1997.
  Includes index.
  ISBN 978-1-84819-133-4 (alk. paper)
  1. Herbs--Therapeutic use. 2. Medicine, Chinese. I. Title.
  RM666.H33H53 2013
  615.3'21--dc23
                            2012040245

British Library Cataloguing in Publication Data
A CIP catalogue record for this book is available from the British Library

ISBN 978 1 84819 133 4
eISBN 978 0 85701 113 8

Printed and bound in Great Britain

CONTENTS

The Growing Interest in Chinese Herbal Medicine

Chinese herbs are parts of a complete medical system that has diagnosed, treated and prevented illness for over 23 centuries. This health care system deals with both physical and mental problems and also strengthens recuperative powers, boosts immunity and the capacity for pleasure, work and activity. It has been working in China for over 2000 years. Today, however, similar treatments are being carried out not just in China, but in such diverse places as the suburbs of Amsterdam, a small village in rural England or a city in the mid-western United States. Chinese herbal medicine has been spreading and growing in popularity.

This popularity has been reflected in increased press and television coverage and the attention of Western doctors. In London, England, for example, the successful use of herbs, especially for skin conditions, has inspired various hospital doctors to examine specific combinations of herbs with the hope of finding the effective 'active ingredients'. In the US there have been numerous studies of the Chinese herbs used for malignant tumours. Indeed, many Western drugs originated in just this way, from the analysis of a successfully used herb. In a more negative vein, you may also have heard of police raids on herbal suppliers where any prescriptions suspected of containing parts of endangered species have been confiscated. And you may have noticed, especially in England, an increasing number of herbal clinics manned by Chinese and run by the government of China.

Are Chinese herbs for you?

This book is for those of you considering Chinese herbal treatment. You may be wondering whether Chinese herbs are right for you. You will have heard that they help a variety of conditions, but will they help you? And what is involved? What are the herbs like? How do you take them? Are they safe? How do they compare with taking drugs? Can you take herbs and take your current medication at the same time? Do you have to have a medical disease before you take herbs?

These are natural questions and this book will give you answers – from the point of view of a Chinese herbalist. I will explain what a visit to a herbalist is like. You will hear about several people who used herbs for a variety of different conditions. You will learn something about the underlying theory, how the herbs are taken and, near the end, we will discuss how you can find and choose a practitioner.

My own experience is as a practitioner of Chinese medicine since 1975. Originally I trained as an acupuncturist, but later learned herbal medicine and now use both together. In Chinese medicine, acupuncture and herbal practice share the same underlying theory and diagnosis, but the means of treatment is different. With some patients I use a combination of herbs and acupuncture and with others I use either acupuncture or herbs on their own. My job in this book is to explain how Chinese herbs can help you.

Acupuncture or herbs?

People often ask whether herbs or acupuncture would be best for them. There is no simple answer to this question. Most practitioners of Chinese medicine – herbalists and acupuncturists – have a view as to the advantages of one over the other and for what complaint. I do not share the beliefs that say one type of treatment is better. I have seen herbs do what acupuncture has failed to do and vice versa. It is probably fair to say that at the moment Chinese herbs have been demonstrated to be more successful with skin diseases and would be preferable in cases of severe inflammation. It is probably also fair to say that anyone whose mind or spirit is disturbed will probably respond more quickly to acupuncture. And I can already hear my colleagues disagreeing.

The difference between the two types of treatment often relates less to the relative effectiveness and more to the other differences.

For example, the nature of the health problem may dictate daily treatment. In that case it would be easier to take herbs, as visiting the practitioner on a daily basis for acupuncture would be difficult and expensive.

Some people love the sensations that occur during an acupuncture treatment; others are needle-phobic. Some people love the taste of their herbal prescription, even love brewing it up; others find the preparation and taste a burden.

Sometimes acupuncture involves more time with the practitioner and a changed state at the time of treatment. Herbs also can be experienced as affecting a person instantly, but less frequently.

The cost of acupuncture treatment is usually the same per treatment. The cost of herbal treatment depends on how often you see the practitioner and the specific herbs and the quantities. So one form of treatment may end up as more economic.

As I said above, I combine the use of herbs and acupuncture and so do many other herbalists. If England is a guide to the practice of Chinese medicine in the West, there are more acupuncturists available, and of the herbalists available many began their career as acupuncturists and therefore can do both. In England, there are roughly ten times as many acupuncturists as herbalists.

The real question, however, is the choice between Western and Chinese medicine. Each has different assumptions about the nature of illness and very different approaches to treatment. As herbs are closer to taking Western drugs, I would like to briefly compare these two.

Chinese herbs and Western medical drugs

Western medicine is committed to objectivity and reproducibility of proof. As a result, it prefers not to deal with the subjectivity of the mind, but instead the physical world, about which there is more agreement. This commitment also leads it to an analytical approach which prefers to break things down to their essential elements, rather than deal with wholes. Traditional Chinese medicine, working with the notion of Organs and Substances, deals more with life as it is experienced. 'Wholes' and subjective judgements have been used throughout. The question is not so much which is right, but which works the best and in what circumstances.

The analytical approach of Western medicine leads it to assume that if a herb works, then there must be some 'part' of it, or ingredient that makes it work. The goal is then to isolate this ingredient, to test it in a trial, and then, if it is proven effective, to use it in its isolated form. If the ingredient can be made in the laboratory, rather than extracted from a plant, so much the better.

One consequence of this chemistry-based approach is that depression or schizophrenia or any problem to do with the mind is thought to have a physical basis and therefore one which can be changed by a drug – if only we can find the right one and get it to the right place. This has been called the 'mechanistic thesis' that has directed so much medical research to the cellular level. Again, there is nothing wrong with this, even though it may seem odd and indeed inappropriate, for example, to try to reduce subjective experiences to chemical events.

As a result of the scientific approach, the Western drug industry has drawn on effective herbs as one of the sources for drugs. It has been estimated that well over one-half of the drugs currently used have been derived from chemicals originally extracted from plants. For example, digoxin, a drug used to strengthen the beat of the heart, was discovered through the Western herbalist's use of foxglove or 'lily of the valley' for much the same use. Ephedrine, which is used for asthma and excessive Phlegm, came from the plant used in Chinese herbal medicine, 'ma huang', or 'ephedra'. As a result of this transference of herbs to drugs, laboratories in the US have systematically looked at all the Substances used by herbalists for tumours in the fight against cancer. So what is the difference between the use of a herb and the use of a drug?

From a patient's point of view, the issues are safety and effectiveness. Is either the drug or herb dangerous and does it work? I will give you some arguments in favour of herbal medicine. But it needs to be said that the line between the two is not absolute and as much depends upon the practitioner prescribing as the pills or formulae prescribed.

The Western testing of a drug shows that it has a certain effect. It does not show or promise that the drug will not have serious side-effects, short term or long term. We now have a cause of illness labelled 'iatrogenesis' meaning caused by medical treatment. The 'illness' in the case of thalidomide was extreme, but in many other cases is serious. The safety problems are sometimes in the drugs and sometimes in the over prescribing. There is clearly a trade-off. A specific drug may help, but is it doing anything else? The increasing numbers of drugs withdrawn from use indicates that safety is always an issue.

Are herbs therefore safe? Not necessarily. Many plants are poisonous and throughout history almost all *materia medicas* (books listing the herbs) have discussed toxicity. When someone first ate a plant, there was no guarantee that it was safe. Mushrooms can be poisonous and, on the other hand, both delicious and nutritious. The current argument for the safety of Chinese herbs is their use for hundreds, and in some cases, thousands of years. The long-term safety-testing for literally thousands of herbs has already been done. It exists in the herbal books, which say how long the herb has been used and give the typical dosages.

Another argument for safety is that the whole plant or parts of a plant is used. The human digestive system is familiar with plant materials and their balance between roughage and active ingredients. An example from Western medicine and herbalism illustrates this. Western medicine discovered that diuretics, which get rid of water by increased urine flow, were depleting the body of potassium. They then added a potassium supplement. Western herbalists use dandelion leaves as a diuretic. These clearly have an active ingredient that increases urine flow. However, dandelion leaves also contain potassium.

Another example. You may remember that aspirins are thought to caused bleeding of the stomach lining and thus the number you can take is limited. A herbalist would use the flowers and leaves of meadowsweet. Meadowsweet has an anti-inflammatory effect because it contains aspirin-like chemicals. But it also contains tannin and mucilage which soothe and protect the lining of the stomach. This is either an argument for the safety of herbs or a demand that isolated ingredients should only be used when more of their side-effects are known.

There are three other factors in favour of Chinese herbs. The first is that within the Chinese *materia medica* there are many tonifying or strengthening herbs. These herbs, like ginseng, encourage the body to function better in a general way. Their use assumes a life force in the body which needs help but not replacing. Very few Western drugs, partly because of their focus on symptoms, have this function.

The second is that when a Western drug is prescribed, it may be the second, third or fourth drug the person is taking. This complicates the issue of side-effects and drug interaction. When a herbalist gives a formula, there are several herbs involved, but they have been used together over and over again.

The third factor is the type of diagnosis that supports the taking of Chinese herbs. A drug will be aimed at a symptom, for example difficulty in breathing. A herb may also be directed at a symptom, but the real basis of diagnosis in Chinese herbs is the condition of the person, not just the breathing difficulty, the headache, or the depression on their own. Herbs are directed at a *pattern of disharmony* (more later) and the prescribing recognises that various symptoms can be caused by different patterns of disharmony and should be treated differently. This is an added safety factor.

A note on vocabulary

Instead of using 'his/her', I will alternate chapters using 'her', then 'his'. I will also begin Chinese terms like Yin and Yang with capital letters. It is obvious with Yin and Yang, but when I write 'Blood' you know I am referring to the Chinese notion of blood which is described in Chapter 3, not our everyday notion of blood. The other ambiguity I have wrestled with is 'Chinese herbalist'. What do you call a Westerner who diagnoses according to Chinese medicine and prescribes Chinese herbs? It is not accurate to call him or her a Chinese herbalist, because he or she is not Chinese. If I call the practitioner a 'herbalist who uses Chinese herbs', that is awkward. If I call him or her just a herbalist, that would include Western herbalists using Western herbs and many others. So what I do is simply refer to a 'herbalist' and in the context of this book this is someone who uses a Chinese diagnosis and prescribes Chinese herbs.

If you are reading this book because of a health problem, or simply because you would like to feel really well more of the time, I wish you the best in finding help from Chinese medicine.

1

How did Chinese Herbal Medicine Develop?

What is unique about Chinese herbal medicine?

Herbs are used throughout the world. Most cultures have a herbal medicine. So what is unique about Chinese herbs?

The answer to this question is not the herbs themselves, but instead the relationship between the herbs, the formulae (groups of herbs) and the diagnosis which underlies their use.

Herbs have been known for thousands of years to have healing properties. The issue is how to deliver exactly the right herbs to a unique individual who is suffering less than perfect health. It is the relationship between the herbs, the formulae and the diagnosis which does this. We need to take these one at a time.

Diagnosis

Diagnosis is expressed in the language of 'patterns of disharmony'. These will be discussed fully in Chapter 3. For the moment, a pattern of disharmony is simply a way of saying which Organ is functioning well or badly, and which overall deficiencies and blockages have developed in the patient's body and mind – independently, or almost independently, of any symptoms.

A patient example might clarify the difference between symptoms and patterns of disharmony. A 30-year-old electrician is restricted to working 10–12 hours a week. He feels heavy and lethargic, in spite of sleeping ten hours a night. His appetite is poor; he eats erratically; and he has almost constant diarrhoea. These are his symptoms; not his diagnosis. After asking questions, looking at his tongue and taking his pulse, the practitioner may say that the electrician has a weak Spleen and Kidney, and as a result has accumulated 'Damp' which is making him feel heavy and lethargic and causing his diarrhoea. ('Damp', you will discover in Chapter 3, is technically called a Pathogenic Factor or something which is blocking or obstructing the normal processes of the body and mind. In this case it is excess Body Fluids.) The herbalist's diagnosis is 'Deficient Spleen and Kidney Yang with Damp' which makes no sense to the electrician, but is the herbalist's diagnosis. 'Deficient Spleen and Kidney Yang with Damp accumulating' is a pattern of disharmony.

There are two crucial effects of diagnosing through patterns of disharmony, rather than symptoms.

One effect is that people with the same symptoms, for example headaches, may have different underlying patterns of disharmony; in one case it may be to do with the Liver, in another with the Stomach. When the herbalist uses the pattern of disharmony to guide the selection of herbs or formulae, rather than just symptoms, the treatment is better adjusted to the patient and will be more successful. Using patterns of disharmony brings not just the symptoms, but the patient into the treatment. Treatment is more successful.

Another effect is that a person can be diagnosed and treated via patterns even though she does not have symptoms. For example, a person may feel unwell, but not really have specific symptoms. This is often the early warning stage of a more serious problem. Such people are frequently told there is nothing wrong with them. They may even be accused of malingering or given anti-depressants. This view ignores their real condition and denies the early warning signs of a later illness. So when the practitioner uses patterns of disharmony, the patient does not have to have specific symptoms in order to ask for help.

Herbs

The development of the herbs consisted of discovering each herb and its specific healing properties. The first discoveries are usually that a herb affects a symptom. Further development of a herb involves two main aspects.

One is how to grow, harvest and process the herb to ensure its greatest effectiveness – something the Chinese have specialised in for centuries. But the other is more crucial. This is to learn to classify the herb in terms of how it affects the patterns of disharmony. For example, it is one thing to say that a herb stops diarrhoea (i.e., affects a symptom); it is another to say that it 'strengthens the Spleen and clears Damp' (i.e., remedies a pattern of disharmony). This is an extraordinary feature of Chinese herbs: they are classified and understood, not just in terms of the symptoms they affect, but by the patterns of disharmony which they remedy.

The importance of this understanding is that the herbs can be used to remedy patterns.

Formulae

A formula is simply several herbs used together, in a harmonious whole. Sometimes one specific herb supplements the effect of another and sometimes one counterbalances the effect of another; but, overall, the formula has a better healing effect than herbs used individually. Other herbal traditions have used herbs together, but the creation of formulae is absolutely basic to Chinese herbal medicine and it provides a more exact healing effect.

Like the herbs, the formulae are classified by their effect on a pattern of disharmony. This extends the benefits described above.

So what is unique to Chinese herbal medicine is this relationship between the herbs, the formulae and the diagnosis. When we speak of the development of Chinese herbal medicine, we speak of all three.

How did it all begin?

A story from ancient China suggests how the benefits of one specific herb were discovered. A farmer is said to have tried to kill a snake by beating it with a hoe. Despite beating the snake severely, the farmer found that the same snake reappeared the following day, hardly the worse for wear. The farmer beat the snake again, and watched as the snake crawled away to some weeds and began to eat them. By the next morning the snake was almost healed, making the farmer curious about the weeds that the snake had eaten.

This observation led to the discovery of what we call 'san qi' or the root of a plant whose botanical name is *Radix Notoginseng*. This plant deals specifically with traumatic injuries because it stops internal or external bleeding, reduces swelling and alleviates pain. Although best known for stopping bleeding, it is still useful when there is no bleeding, but simply swelling and bruising. Today, it is used in decoctions (the liquid left over when the herb is boiled in water), which are drunk, or pills which are eaten or swallowed, or powders and salves which are applied externally.

Imagine the importance of this herb to an army fighting hand to hand and suffering many traumatic injuries. It was the first-aid kit of ancient China. As a result, early Chinese soldiers called it 'Gold-no-trade'. What they meant, of course, was that their supply of san qi was not to be traded – even for gold.

This method of discovery still goes on. In a more modern setting, many people know that when your leg has been severely irritated by stinging nettles, that the nearby burdock leaves, when rubbed on the skin, relieve the sting. A close-to-hand, simple example of how we discover the healing effect of plants.

It is worth noting that when someone makes such a discovery, what they learn is that the herb affects a symptom, not a pattern of disharmony.

When was this happening? Scholars believe that Chinese herbal medicine goes back at least 5000 years, long before recorded history. At this time, medicine was practised by shamans. A shaman is person who makes a link between the natural and supernatural worlds – between our world and that of the gods and goddesses. This link, often made by the shaman entering a trance or unusual internal state, explains the shaman's deeper and more god-like understanding.

One of the greatest shamans was a legendary emperor called Shen Nong. He was worshipped at the beginning of the agricultural year so that the crops might be plentiful and he is also the father of herbal medicine. He was thought to have lived around 3494 BC and was said, by the famous historians of the Han dynasty (around the birth of Christ), to have tested the medicinal value of many herbs by taking them himself.

This taking of herbs to test them refers to another source of information about herbs. This source is a person with greater than normal sensitivity who eats the herb and then determines that it is, for example, warming rather than cooling, or affects the heart rather than the stomach or kidneys, or makes the blood flow more smoothly, and so on. Shen Nong is reported to have done this and symbolically represents all those shamans through the centuries who accessed the wisdom of plants. Without doubt, this has been an important source of information.

At the time of Shen Nong, there were no written records and superstition was mixed together with the medicine. The only written records remaining are tortoise shells with prayers for the sick carved on them. So the herbal knowledge of Shen Nong was passed down, by word of mouth, from one generation to the next and from shaman to shaman. It was probably more than 2000 years, around 1500 BC, before the original observations of Shen Nong were actually written down.

One clue as to how 'medicine' fared during that time was found in 1973. Eleven medical texts were excavated from a burial tomb in Hunan province in China. The burial occurred in 168 BC, but the texts, written on silk, bamboo and wooden strips, are dated at around 900 BC. Several of these refer to herbal medicine and they tell us several features of its state at that time.

The first is that the process of a naturalistic diagnosis, prior to the third century BC, was not advanced. Instead of a scientific process of trial and observation, much magic and superstition was involved. There was no reference yet to patterns of disharmony; the formulae were used on the basis of symptoms. The texts in the burial tomb imply that disease is a result of the influence of malevolent spirits, ghosts and demons which are to be repelled, not just with herbal prescriptions, but incantations, rituals and spells devised by the 'doctor'. So the herbs and formulae developed over

2000 or more years were used, but were empowered by the words and magic of the shaman-doctor.

The second feature of the use of herbs from Shen Nong down to 300 BC is that 242 medicinal Substances were mentioned. The majority of these were from the vegetable kingdom – herbaceous and woody Substances, grains, fruits, roots and vegetables – but some were animal parts and some minerals. The kudzu vine, used today for dysentery, was mentioned in these texts. Ginger as a warming herb was also mentioned.

The third feature is that the Substances were mainly used in formulae or groups of herbs and these formulae were linked to specific health problems. Many of these were inflammations, for example of the skin or urinary tract, and many were traumatic issues such as wounds, injuries, hernias and bites. The formulae would be pre-made and then kept where they would be needed. So, although diagnosis through patterns of disharmony was not developed, the use of herbs in formulae was.

This is the story up to around 200 BC. What was the next big step?

The next big step

The next major development of Chinese herbal medicine was the publication, around 200 BC, of a book called the *Nei Jing* (pronounced Nay Jing). This book was a discussion between the Yellow Emperor and his doctor Chi Po. The *Nei Jing* made several significant changes.

The first was the development of diagnosis. Somewhere in the few hundred years before the publication of the *Nei Jing*, remarkable progress had been made in the way of describing disease. The type of diagnosis referred to earlier was written down at that time.

A distinction was made between the 'root' of a 'disease' and its manifestation. In the example of the electrician, the manifestation of the disease is the lethargy and diarrhoea; the root of the disease is the 'Spleen and Kidney Deficiency leading to Damp'. The principle was established in the *Nei Jing* that similar symptoms could have different roots, and this principle changes medicine enormously. The doctor can directly treat a symptom, but he or she can also treat the root and thereby have a wider, more systemic effect. The 'root' of a disease is a pattern of disharmony.

The second change indicated in the *Nei Jing* was the naturalistic attitude to medical knowledge. This meant that less emphasis was placed on superstition and magic and more on written records, experiment and observation. Devils and spirits as causes of disease were diminished in importance. At that time the belief emerged that the basic laws of nature which governed the lowest creatures also governed the higher ones. Man, or woman, was not separate from nature or the cosmos: the laws governing one govern all.

The third change noted in the *Nei Jing* was the importance attached to exercise and proper diet. As causes of disease, less weight was given to malevolent spirits and more to diet and exercise. The importance of diet, particularly, is significant, as we will see later that there is only a degree of difference between good diet and taking herbs to cure an illness.

These changes in the *Nei Jing* were echoed by other changes in society and language. Somewhere in the century before Christ, the word 'yao', meaning medicine, appeared in the Chinese language. Around the same time 'yi' meaning doctor also appeared. After 'yi' and 'yao', 'ben cao' meaning herbal medicine began to be used. So medicine and herbal doctors became part of the structure of society.

Development after the Nei Jing

Herbal medicine developed more quickly after the *Nei Jing*. The development from then to today is best described by referring to selected great books and doctors.

In the century before Christ, and some time after the publication of the *Nei Jing*, a book was published called *The Divine Husbandman's Classic of Herbal Medicine*. The 'Divine Husbandman' was, of course, Shen Nong. Some 3000 years after he was supposed to have lived, this book detailed the herbs from his time and the ones developed in the intervening period. The book listed 365 Substances, most of them plants.

The herbs or Substances were classified as superior, average and inferior. This ranking was the beginning of determining the functions of herbs according to the understanding in the *Nei Jing*. One hundred and twenty were classified as superior and this meant that they were not toxic and, more important, that they produced a strengthening effect. One of the superior herbs was ginseng which is acknowledged today as one of the main strengthening Substances. The inferior herbs were more toxic and were often used to expel Substances from the body.

This distinction between strengthening and expelling matches the notion of some illness being based on an empty condition and some being based on a full condition. In the former, the patient, or more specifically an Organ or Substance of the patient, requires strengthening; in the latter the patient is required to get rid of something, for example Phlegm stuck in the lungs. So the herbal repertoire was becoming classified in such a way as to match the understanding of disease in the *Nei Jing*.

The Divine Husbandman's Classic also classified herbs by taste and temperature and we will discuss this more fully in Chapter 5.

Around 200 AD, another key figure emerged. A herbal practitioner called Zhang, who lived in the coldest part of China, saw two-thirds of his family killed off by diseases which started off by exposure to cold. Zhang became a doctor and studied how these cold-induced diseases progressed. He detailed the stages of the illness and developed a system of classification to say how far the illness had penetrated and which herbs and formulae should be used. He also formulated the principle that herbs should be prescribed based on the overall understanding of the patient's signs and symptoms, not just symptoms. As a result, he produced the first clinical manual for herbs and his book, the *Shang Han Lun* is still a textbook today and many of the formulae that Zhang wrote down are still in use.

As well as the effect of the herb being understood better, more and more Substances came into use. The number of Substances used for medicinal purposes grew from the 365 in *The Divine Husbandman's Classic of Herbal Medicine*. The following table gives the numbers of plants or Substances in use at specific dates.

Date	Numbers of herbs and Substances recorded
100 BC	365
659 AD	844
1108 AD	1558
1596 AD	1892
1977 AD	5767

Another important development was the concept of preventing an illness before it appeared. This idea arose early in Chinese medicine. One famous practitioner, Qin Yueren (pronounced Chin-your-en), who lived 407–310 BC, has a story told about him.

Upon visiting the King, Qin explained that his lordship was ill, but the disease at the moment was only affecting the surface of the body. If precautions were not taken, however, the illness would become worse. The King proclaimed that he was well and took no notice. This interchange was repeated three times. Each time Qin described the illness going deeper: from the skin to the muscles to the intestines and stomach. Each time the King brushed Qin aside. The final time, Qin avoided the King and the King asked what was wrong. Qin was forced to explain that at each stage a disease becomes more difficult to cure. Now that it had reached the bones, it was impossible to change. Five days later the King was ill and called for Qin who could not be found. Seven days later the King died.

The story may sound dramatic, but it illustrates an important understanding of Chinese medicine. Being able to diagnose using more than just symptoms allows treatment to occur before an illness has fully developed.

One famous doctor, Sun Simiao who lived 581–682 AD, was very influential in promoting this idea. Sun was known as the 'King of Herbal Formulae' and wrote a book, drawing on previous authors, entitled *Formulae of a Thousand Ducats of Gold*. He is credited with the following quote: 'Superior treatment consists of dealing with an illness before it appears, mediocre treatment consists of curing an illness on the point of revealing itself; inferior treatment consists of curing the illness once it has manifested itself.'

If you think about this quote, you have to conclude that very few doctors or patients follow the implicit recommendation.

Associated with this idea is that of health, longevity and spirituality being connected. The Daoists fostered the idea of becoming an 'immortal' which in part meant living a long life and in part meant developing oneself in a spiritual sense.

This lead to a demand being put on herbalists in particular to produce an elixir of immortality. Certain emperors are thought to have died from overdosing on certain toxic herbs which they believed were going to make them live forever.

One of the signs of development is that more distinctions are made and then recorded. In 600 AD a book was published giving much better quality of information about the herbs. It gave information for each Substance on the taste, temperature, toxicity, primary clinical application, processing and preparation and herbal combinations, which show how one herb works well with another herb to produce certain results.

In the seventeenth century, more herbs were used and many doctors had developed formulae (or groups of herbs) and linked these not just to symptoms, but to the underlying patterns of disharmony. A re-examination occurred at this time and two schools of thought arose as to how a formula should be constructed.

One school opted for simplicity and the other for greater complexity. The former school preferred the classical formulae of Zhang who wrote the treatise on cold-induced diseases. His formulae contained fewer herbs with larger quantities of each herb. The other school used more herbs in a formula with smaller quantities of each herb.

The issue here is not which school was correct, but more that the construction of a formula had been seriously studied from the time of Zhang (100 AD) and much practical testing had been carried out. Evidence of these two tendencies – fewer herbs and larger quantities and more herbs and smaller quantities – still exists in the work of herbalists today.

From 1850 onwards, when Western medicine was introduced into China, attention was less focused on the development of herbal medicine. This situation was changed from 1949 when Mao Ze Dong encouraged the reawakening of traditional medicine and its integration with Western medicine. What is currently called TCM in the West – meaning, of course, traditional Chinese medicine – was the systematisation of a varied set of traditional medical practices. Today, there are herbal clinics in many integrated hospitals and some hospitals which specialise in only herbal treatment.

Having considered how herbs, formulae and patterns of disharmony developed, we now can look at what a visit to a herbalist might include.

2

What is it Like to Visit a Herbalist and Take Herbs?

People who are considering herbal treatment often wonder what it would be like to visit a herbalist. Herbalists, of course, vary a lot and visiting one might seem very different from another. But essentially they are going through a similar process and you may appreciate an overview.

So what is the herbalist looking for?

The herbalist starts off seeking a diagnosis and the diagnosis guides what happens during the first consultation.

The diagnosis is phrased in terms of 'patterns of disharmony' which we will discuss more fully in Chapter 3. A pattern of disharmony is a way of saying that someone's energy is deficient, disturbed or blocked in a certain way; and the herbalist's job is to discover the pattern and help to restore a normal balance. The patterns are recognised by a combination of symptoms, mental states, non-verbal behaviour, physiological signs and a reading of both the tongue and pulse. So, effectively, the herbalist is gathering these signs and symptoms during the consultation and at the same time putting the patterns together as he goes along. Once he has the patterns, the decision about the herbs is almost made.

To do this, most herbalists will carry out the following steps, but there is essentially no right or correct order.

What is your complaint?

You will be asked what problem or complaint you would like to change with Chinese herbs. Most people consulting a herbalist have a 'complaint', but the notion is relative. People sometimes take a problem to the doctor and, after tests, the doctor says that there is nothing wrong. This can lead to confusion. For example, people can say 'I feel bad, but I am told there is nothing wrong with me; maybe it's all in my mind,' and so on.

Simply not feeling well is a sufficient complaint for the herbalist. It is his job to ferret out and understand why you are not feeling well. He will address your complaint and it may well be an important pointer to the diagnosis. But, whatever you say, the herbalist will be forming a diagnosis which in his understanding explains the problems you have and will improve your health.

Whatever your complaint, you will be asked several questions about it. Some of the key questions are the following:

- What are the details of your complaint? For example, if you are suffering, for example, from pain or depression, how do you describe it, where is it, does it come and go, how intense is it, what can you not do as a result of it?

- What makes it worse or better? For example, what are the effects of specific foods, rest, activity, time of day, climate, work or family stress?

- How long have you had this problem, and did it come on slowly or rapidly?

- What was happening at the time for it to occur?

- Are there any accompanying symptoms that typically precede or co-exist with this problem?

- What have you done already? Are you currently taking any medication?

What else will the herbalist ask?

The herbalist will question many other aspects of how your body and mind are functioning. He is still collecting the ingredients of the 'patterns' and needs to be thorough in order not to misdiagnose you.

Traditionally, there were said to be ten main areas to question, but the following will give a good idea of the questions you might be asked.

Chills and fevers

These cover what happens when you get an infection or cold. When someone feels cold and cannot get warm, even by wrapping up and piling on the blankets, this indicates that certain herbs should be used. If the 'cold' is predominantly a hot or dry one, other herbs will be used. But generally, even when the patient has no infection, the patient's reaction to cold and heat will be questioned as it often reflects, from the herbalist's point of view, something of your state of health. Many people who desperately feel the cold, but that is not their complaint, are delighted after treatment to find that they are less affected by the cold. You will also be asked about your predisposition to catch colds.

Sweating

The tendencies for a person to wake up sweating or to sweat with little exertion during the day are important for

Women's issues

Women will be asked a special set of questions around menstruation, premenstrual behaviour, discharges, pregnancy and childbirth. Although there may be no complaints in any of these areas, the history, for example of childbirths, and the current information as to what happens pre-period, is often important in confirming 'patterns' which are mainly affecting other areas.

History

In any of the above areas where a symptom comes up, the herbalist will probably ask about the history of the symptom. Also, in a more general way, he will ask about your medical history, focusing more on any serious past medical problems.

Children

Children are excellent subjects for herbal medicine. Depending upon age, the questioning approach will vary. Often many of the above areas will be best answered either by the parent or the child and parent together.

Lifestyle

You will also be asked about your living situation, relationships, family, patterns of work, rest and exercise. For centuries, the Chinese have valued good health and living to an old age. They have observed what leads to these and have numerous rules of thumb to do with maintaining health and living long. Your herbalist will want to know whether your lifestyle is affecting your health positively or negatively. He may make recommendations for improvement.

Taking the pulse and observing the tongue

The herbalist will feel your pulse and look at your tongue. These are two very old methods of diagnosis. Pulse and tongue signs are some of the most important indicators that go to make up a 'pattern'.

Pulse

The herbalist will feel your pulse on both wrists and in three positions on each wrist. He is feeling for different qualities, one of which is the number of beats per minute, just as your doctor would record. The other qualities include such factors as the strength or weakness of the pulse, its width or thinness, whether it is felt on the surface or only on deeper pressure, whether there are any irregularities and what the 'shape' of the beat feels like. There are 15 basic pulse qualities and 28 in total. They all have a clinical significance and are strong pointers to the final diagnosis. They take considerable experience to feel accurately.

Tongue

Tongue characteristics are also important. You will be asked to stick your tongue out in a comfortable way. Leaving your tongue out too long can change some of its characteristics, so you will probably be asked to leave it out only for a matter of seconds, but repeat the process a few times. The herbalist will be looking at the tongue body – shape, colour and cracks – and the tongue coating – thickness, colour and location. The tongue, like the pulse, provides vital information for the diagnosis. To know what a 'normal' tongue looks like is the starting point, and this requires countless observations.

Why are the pulse and tongue so important? Take an example. Suppose the patient is a woman entering menopause who is feeling abnormally hot, having difficulty sleeping and experiencing itchy skin. She could be more Yin Deficient or she could be more Blood Deficient. In the former case the tongue body will be red; in the latter, pale. The tongue helps decide and the herbs will differ. Or suppose the patient has attacks of difficult breathing with very little wheezing. The problem could be coming more from the Liver or more from the Lungs and Kidney. In the former case the pulse will be 'wiry' (tight like a guitar string), in the latter 'weak' and 'deep', especially in two of the six positions. The more experienced the herbalist, the more reliance placed on pulse and tongue.

Observation throughout your visit

One thing you may not notice your herbalist doing is observing you carefully throughout the visit. There are many 'signs' which a Western doctor might ignore, but which Chinese medicine says are indications of the underlying patterns. Each pattern of disharmony will have various aspects of a person associated with it. For example, it is part of some Blood Deficiency patterns that the person will be more 'jumpy' and 'easily startled'. Your herbalist will be paying attention to the subtleties of your behaviour as well as what you are saying. More about these in Chapter 3.

Near the end of the first visit, the herbalist will be putting all the information together and coming up with a diagnosis. He will decide on the right herbs for you and also how you should take them. What are the choices here?

How do you take the herbs?

Decoctions, pills, powders and tinctures are the main options and there are many considerations in deciding which is best. We will look at each of these and ask: what are they, how are they prepared and what are the advantages?

Decoctions

A decoction is what you get when dried herbs are put into a saucepan, covered in water and the water is simmered for 20 to 30 minutes. Some of the water evaporates, but what is left contains the formula's active ingredients. This liquid is poured off, usually through a sieve, and then drunk. Sometimes the process is repeated with the same herbs. The word for the liquid in Chinese is 'tang' and it is translated both as 'decoction' or 'soup'.

How do you get the Substances in the first place? Your herbalist may keep the dried herbs himself. In this case he will measure out the correct amount of each ingredient and put the mixture in a small paper bag or wrap it in a sheet of paper similar to that used in a fish and chip shop. Alternatively, the prescription is sent to a herbal pharmacy which carry out the same process.

How many bags and how often do you use each? This varies. You may, for example, get five bags, each of which is simmered twice and lasts for two days. So the five bags last for ten days. You may use the herbs in one bag twice, but drink both in one day. You may be given only a few bags because the herbalist thinks that the effect will be quick and the formula will need to change. You may be given more because the problem is chronic and it is safe to proceed with the same herbs for a longer time. There are many variations here. They arise out of the herbalist's diagnosis and depend upon whether your condition requires clearing or strengthening, is severe or less so, and is acute or chronic.

Decoctions have certain advantages. The active ingredients are rapidly absorbed in the stomach and their effects can be felt almost immediately. They are therefore good for acute problems. They are also easily modified by the practitioner so that, if a formula needs to be created just for you, the decoction is a good option.

On the other hand, being custom made, decoctions take time to prepare and can be more expensive. Additionally, some patients find the decocting process too difficult and the taste of the decocted herbs unpleasant. This supposed 'bad taste' of Chinese herbs is somewhat exaggerated. Many patients say they love the taste of their decoction and feel very good drinking it. Admittedly, there is an objective side to taste. A bitter-tasting, heat-clearing formula will not be actively liked by many people, while a sweeter Qi tonifying one will often be enjoyed.

Pills

Another alternative is pills. Most pills are manufactured in China but they are increasingly made in the United States and Europe with imported herbs. Substances are ground into a fine powder and then some binding agent is added. The binding agent varies. It can be honey, beeswax, sesame oil, water, vinegar, wine, rice or wheat flour paste or a combination of these. The mixture is shaped into pills and dried for easy handling and storage.

Another method is to make a large decoction and then, using heat, to concentrate the decoction to a thick paste. Pills are then formed with a binder or filler. Pills made from decoctions are often the most concentrated.

Pills come in various sizes. The typical ones from China are relatively small, 2–5mm in diameter. For anyone used to taking Western doctor's pills, the number of herbals pills seems excessive. But the principle is different. A Western drug is mainly the active ingredients while the herbal pills are mainly ground herbs.

Pills need to be dissolved in the stomach. For this reason the absorption rate is relatively slow and the therapeutic effects prolonged. If the purpose of the formula is not acute, then pills are often ideal.

Like the dried herbs, your herbalists may have the pills in his surgery or ask you to get them from a herbal supplier. The pills will be in glass or plastic containers or blister packs. Again, you will be told how many to take, how often and at what time of day.

Aside from the advantage of slow absorption, pills can easily be stored and carried around. Whereas it would be difficult to take your decoction to work, taking a few pills is simple. Also, if you are prone to colds and these are easily identified as typically Wind-Cold or Wind-Heat, then you can have the appropriate remedy in pill form at home ready to take. Pills also tend to be less expensive.

Powders and granules

Powders have two sources. Sometimes they are simply the Substances of the formula ground to a very fine powder. Sometimes they are the dried residue of a decoction made into a powder. The latter powder is more concentrated. Whichever way the powder is made, it is supplied in plastic containers. You often also get a 5ml spoon for easy measuring.

Your herbalist may have the powders in stock, but, more likely, they will be purchased from a herbal pharmacy.

The powder can be taken in different ways. Frequently it is mixed with water. The powder can be put in a cup and hot water poured in, as you would make a cup of instant coffee. Or the powder can be put in a saucepan and boiled with a small amount of water and then poured into a cup. Alternatively, the powder can be taken directly, but it is extremely dry and even a small amount is hard to swallow. For this reason, powdered formulae are often put in gelatinous capsules for easier swallowing. There is one formula used for reviving a patient from a coma that can be blown into the mouth or nose.

One advantage of powders is their greatly increased surface area and therefore rapid absorption. They are probably a little more slowly absorbed than a decoction, but faster acting then pills. Like pills, they are easily stored, but somewhat less easy to carry around, and if stored too long after opening, will solidify. Like decoctions, they can be custom formulated.

Powders may also be used externally. They can be put directly on the skin or first mixed with some medium such as alcohol, vinegar, sesame oil, or water to form a paste, which in turn is applied to the skin. Plasters have been used from the beginning of herbal medicine. The powdered herbs were made into a paste, put on a cloth or animal skin that was folded over and allowed to dry. When used, the plaster was warmed and softened and then applied to the skin. Today, there are ready-made plasters using adhesive strips and sealed plastic bags to preserve the active ingredients. As an example, one of these contains mainly Blood moving herbs. You peel off a plastic covering and then stick the adhesive strip to an area where there is pain, strain or injury. Blood moving herbs are then in close contact with the skin and quickly penetrate the subcutaneous tissue. This can be a very effective way of helping an injury to heal or dissipating rheumatic or arthritic pain.

Granules are a modern variation on powders. They resemble freeze-dried as opposed to powdered coffee. They begin as a decoction, which is made in the factory and not in your kitchen. It is simmered to a thick, concentrated syrup to which a paste is added. The paste is made from starch or the ground-up dregs of the decoction process. The syrup and paste mixture is then processed through a series of sieves and rollers and the final product dried into granules. It is thought that granules have a longer shelf life, are quickly absorbed and are very concentrated. Otherwise they are like powders.

Tinctures

Tinctures are formed by soaking the herbs in rice wine or other spirits, using the alcohol as a solvent. Sometimes the resulting fluid, which contains the active ingredients and some alcohol, is further processed by heating in order to evaporate off some of the solvent. Your herbalist will know the concentration of any tinctures and will set your dosage accordingly. Tinctures are taken by the teaspoonful or by the drop and are easy to take and easy to absorb.

These are the various ways to take your herbs. If it seems confusing, there is no need to worry. Your herbal practitioner will select a way that is right for you.

What happens after I take the herbs?

After arranging for you to take the herbs, the herbalist will ask you to visit again. The gap will depend on how soon you are expected to respond. At the next visit you will report on your progress and your herbalist will take your pulses, look at your tongue, ask some of the same questions and again observe you carefully. Effectively, he is monitoring changes and furthering the diagnosis.

There are various possibilities at this stage. If you are progressing well, you may be asked to continue with the same herbs. On the other hand, if parts of your problem have been fully resolved, the herbs may be changed. If you were, for example, to have caught a cold, additional herbs may be added to address this problem in the short term.

The numbers of visits and the numbers of times the herbs are changed depends, of course, on the individual. Some examples are discussed in Chapter 4 on patients.

You now have some idea what a visit to the herbalist includes. We will now turn to the underlying theory of Chinese medicine.

3

Chinese Medical Theory

We have discussed the development of Chinese herbal medicine and considered a visit to a herbalist. In both cases, reference was made to 'patterns of disharmony'. It is time now to examine more thoroughly these patterns of disharmony and the theory which underlies them.

Patterns of disharmony

Chinese medical diagnosis is expressed in 'patterns of disharmony' and patterns are recognised through 'signs' and 'symptoms'.

Signs are something that the herbalist can observe, like a pale dull colour of your face, a rapid pulse rate, a purple tongue or behaviour which is restless and agitated. Symptoms, on the other hand, are the things we report to the herbalist and, sometimes, but not always, what we might be complaining about. For instance, tiredness, a cough, feeling depressed and constipation are all symptoms. In a pattern, the signs and symptoms hang together. The easiest way to understand a pattern is to take an example.

One commonly occurring pattern is labelled 'Heart Blood Deficient'. Here are the typical signs and symptoms of this pattern.

HEART BLOOD DEFICIENCY

Symptoms	Signs
Feeling the heart beating without exertion; slight dizziness; difficulty in getting off to sleep; sleeping lightly; poor memory and absent-mindedness; feeling anxious; being easily startled, for example when the phone rings.	Pale, dull face; pale lips and nails; state of anxiety; hypersensitivity to outside stimuli. Pulse: Choppy or thin. Tongue: Pale, thin, and slightly dry.

A person can have Heart Blood Deficiency (or any pattern) to a greater or lesser degree. She need not have all the symptoms, but some of them are more important than others. In the case of Heart Blood Deficiency, poor sleep and absent-mindedness are symptoms of greater significance. Amongst the signs, the pale dull face, the pale and dry tongue and the choppy pulse are more significant. Pulse and tongue characteristics are always important.

How many patterns are there? There is no exact answer to this question. Patterns overlap and throughout the ages have been described with slightly different boundaries. But your herbalist will be working with a repertoire of 75 basic patterns and many variations on each of these.

How many patterns will a patient have? That depends, of course, on the state of the patient's health. It may be anywhere from one to several, although with several patterns some of these will be more important and require attention first. 'More important' refers to the intensity of the pattern. A person can be very mildly Heart Blood Deficient or severely so. The judgement as to the intensity of the pattern is therefore important in choosing the correct herbs and the correct dosage.

The question now is 'How do patterns relate to Chinese medical theory?' Patterns have labels. The example above was called Heart Blood Deficient. The language of the label comes from four broad categories of theory. These are Yin and Yang, Substances, Organs and Pathogenic Factors. These are the building blocks of patterns.

A simple view of the theory

Yin/Yang together are like a net through which all the elements of theory pass. Any Organ, Substance or Pathogenic Factor will be either more Yin or more Yang and either Yin or Yang relative to any other. Thus, Yin and Yang become an organising principle for theory as well as part of the theory itself.

On the other hand, the Organs, Substances and Pathogenic Factors are three basic categories. The Organs, such as the Heart, Kidneys or Lungs, are the factories that produce the material of life. The Substances, which are the various grades of the material of life, are a product of the Organs. The Pathogenic Factors are the dirt in the machine – the material which is stopping the factories and the materials of life from functioning at their best.

So Organs can underfunction. Substances can be in short supply, disturbed or stagnating. Pathogenic Factors obstruct and generally lower the ability of an Organ or Substance to do its job. As a result, treatment frequently strengthens Organs, supports and eases the Substances and expels the Pathogenic Factors.

With this overview in mind, let us look first at Yin and Yang.

Yin and Yang

The Chinese have seen the world through the concepts of Yin and Ying for several thousand years. Yin and Yang were popularised through a school called the Yin-Yang School which flourished around 2–300 BC. The meaning of Yin and Yang is contained in the characters used to represent them.

The Chinese character for Yang depicts the sunny side of a hill; the character for Yin, the shady side of a hill. The hill, sun and shade image is full of meaning. As well as being opposites, the shady and sunny sides are inseparable – you can't have one without the other. In addition, sun and shade affect each other: increase the sun and you diminish the shade and vice versa. Sun and shade also raise the issue of balance: all sun and no shade leads to death; so does all shade and no sun. This Yin/Yang understanding underlies much of Chinese thought.

To understand how Yin and Yang are used medically we need to extend the notions of the sunny and shady side of the hill.

Yang	Yin
Sunny side of hill	Shady side of hill
Fire	Water
Hot	Cold
Restless	Quiet
Dry	Wet
Rapid	Slow
Outward moving	Inward moving
Restless, insomnia	Sleepy, lethargic
Hot limbs and body	Cold limbs and body
Loud voice, talks a lot	Weak voice, dislikes talking
Lies stretched out	Lies curled up

The analysis of Yin and Yang opposites is infinite. Behind it is the belief that any of the events to do with health and illness can be understood as having two aspects, Yin and Yang, which are to a greater or lesser degree in balance.

We can illustrate this thinking with two important patterns: Yang Deficiency and Yin Deficiency. Someone who is 'Yang Deficient' is short on Yang energy, which is warming, moving and outgoing. Someone who is 'Yin Deficient' is short on Yin energy, which is cooling, still and inward moving.

So the Yang Deficient person has cold limbs, frequently feels chilly, tends to be lethargic and sleepy and is reluctant to get up and go. This person also has a pale face, a pale swollen tongue and a deep and weak pulse.

By contrast, the Yin Deficient person feels warmer to the touch, feels the cold much less, tends to be restless and frequently on the go, and finds it harder to relax and quietly contemplate by closing her eyes and looking inward. This person has red cheeks, a red tongue with little tongue coating, and a floating, more rapid pulse. So the Yin Deficient person and the Yang Deficient person are different and have different herbal needs.

The next building block of the patterns is Substances.

Substances

Substances are what the herbal practitioner would say a person is made up of. They are the 'material' of the body, mind and spirit, and they enable the herbalist to talk about a person in several useful ways.

So what are these Substances? There are five: Shen, Qi, Jing, Blood and Body Fluids. The following table indicates what each does.

Substance	Meaning
Shen	Mind/Spirit: to do with sleep, consciousness, memory, thinking and spirit
Qi	Energy: the body and mind's ability to move and transform, keep warm
Jing	Inherited constitutional energy: sets limits to health
Blood	Nourishes and moistens the various parts of the body, and holds or 'roots' the Mind or Shen
Body Fluids	For example, saliva, synovial fluid, sweat, etc.: moisten and cool

Substances are often abbreviated to three – Jing, Qi and Shen – and these are called the Three Treasures to indicate their value to us and to suggest the importance of our looking after them.

The herbalist uses Substances to diagnose – as part of the patterns. The question in the back of her mind is 'How are this person's Substances? How is their Qi and how is their Blood and how is their Shen?' Behind this question is the fact that each Substance has one or more ways of being out of balance. Let us look first at the Shen.

Shen or Mind/Spirit

Shen can be out of balance in three ways: it can be deficient, disturbed and obstructed. How would you know?

Shen governs several functions: memory, consciousness, thought and sleep. For this reason, Shen symptoms are mainly mental, including such things as absent-mindedness, lapses in consciousness, dull and poorly directed thinking and waking frequently in the night.

Shen imbalance	Typical signs and symptoms
Shen Deficiency	Mental dullness, lack of spirit, lethargy, chronic sadness, lack of vitality
Shen Disturbance	Insomnia, dream-disturbed sleep, easily startled, absent-mindedness, anxiety
Obstructed Shen	Lapses of consciousness, inappropriate crying and laughing, incoherent speech, muttering to self, mental depression or dullness

Deficient Shen, for example, includes mental dullness, lack of vitality and chronic sadness. Many people could identify with these when they say they are depressed or feeling sad. For the herbalist, if a patient says 'I'm depressed', it may well be that they are describing Deficient Shen.

Disturbed Shen is slightly different and includes such symptoms as being chronically anxious, sleeping lightly, and being easily startled. Disturbed Shen comes about when another Substance, the Blood, is deficient. We will discuss Blood below, but as an example, a woman who loses much blood giving birth, or who has had prolonged heavy periods, will easily become Blood Deficient. When the Blood is deficient, the Shen has no root and the mind is easily disturbed. Some women, who are only a little Blood Deficient, will notice that around period time, just before and just after, that some of the same symptoms appear. Depression after giving birth, especially when the birth involved considerable bleeding, is usually understood this way.

Obstructed Shen is often the category of serious mental illnesses. The Chinese speak of the heart as having 'openings'. These openings need to be clear and open for the Mind or Spirit to function well. If the 'openings of the Heart' become obstructed, then the energy and Shen cannot move freely and the mind is restricted. The Chinese knew of the brain, but often spoke as if the mind was located in the heart. Typical symptoms of Obstructed Shen are bipolar disorder and schizophrenia, which involve big variations and inconsistencies in consciousness and thinking.

The quickest way to assess someone's Shen is by the 'sparkle' in their eyes (this is the quickest way, not necessarily the complete way). Assessing sparkle would not be considered 'scientific' in the Western medical context. Nevertheless, the herbalist will have observed 'sparkle' countless times and be able to make an early diagnosis based on this observation alone.

Qi or energy

'Qi' is not an easy word to translate. The best translation is 'energy', but this only gives a rough indication. The two main imbalances of Qi are Qi Deficiency and Qi Stagnation. What are the key signs and symptoms?

Qi imbalance	Typical signs and symptoms
Qi Deficiency	Chronic tiredness, poor appetite, loose bowels, feelings of the limbs and body being heavy, weakness of muscles, prolapses, bleeding, weak pulse, pale tongue
Qi Stagnation	Symptoms that come and go (usually with emotional stress), chronic irritability, lump in throat, stuffiness in the chest, indigestion of various sorts, flatulence, masses which come and go, wiry pulse

The Chinese say that the Qi of the human has several functions.

- Qi enables us to *move*: movement in the sense of walking, taking a breath, moving our bowels, laughing, singing or dancing.

- Qi enables us to *transform*: particularly in the sense of changing food and drink into new flesh and blood and energy.

- Qi *protects*: our ability to ward off colds and flu is a function of good Qi.

- Qi *warms*: feeling chronically cold and hating winter comes from Deficient Qi.

- Qi *holds* the blood in the blood vessels: some sorts of bleeding, especially lingering post-period bleeding, is due to deficiency of Qi.

Overall the Qi enables us to move, to transform food, to ward off colds and infections, to keep warm, and to hold the blood in our blood vessels. Chronic deficiency of Qi will lead to any of those functions being weak, resulting in such symptoms as poor digestion, tiredness, frequent colds, chilliness, and a chronic and scanty bleeding typical of the spotting that can occur when the normal menstrual flow stops. These are Qi Deficiency symptoms.

Qi Stagnation is the second important imbalance of Qi, and is somewhat more elusive. There are two notions of Qi Stagnation.

In a specific, physical sense, a patient might have Qi Stagnation after a physical injury. An ankle is twisted playing football or a back sprained by lifting. The Chinese call the effect of the injury 'Qi and Blood Stagnation', because, temporarily, the energy and Blood needed to heal the muscles and tendons is blocked. In the West, we prescribe pain killers and rest. Chinese herbal medicine would use herbs which move the Qi and Blood, thus relieving the Stagnation. These herbs accelerate the healing process.

Qi Stagnation also occurs in a more general way. In this case the Qi may be adequate – no Qi Deficiency – but it is flowing irregularly. Sometimes it is there; sometimes it isn't. Symptoms come and go; periods are irregular; digestion is good one day, bad another. The bowels are loose one day, then constipated the next. One of the key signs is the coming and going of symptoms – often, the patient will say, with no rhyme or reason. The coming and going, however, is frequently associated with frustration and repressed irritability or failure to express feelings.

Chronic Qi Stagnation often leads to pain and the formation of lumps, both of which will come and go. A principle of Chinese medicine is that pain usually involves obstruction and Qi Stagnation is an obstruction. For example, Qi Stagnation easily increases just before a period, and some women will often experience irritability, increase in breast lumps or soreness of the breasts, and lower abdomen pain at that time. Chronic obstruction caused by Qi Stagnation leads to parts of the body being deprived of nourishment and, in the long term, is often a factor in cancer.

The next Substance to consider is Jing.

Jing or constitutional energy

Jing is sometimes translated as 'Essence', a term which implies its utmost fundamental nature. Jing gives the person an ability to grow, develop and reproduce. Jing is considered to have only one imbalance: deficiency. What symptoms would be present when Jing is deficient?

Jing imbalance	Typical signs and symptoms
Jing Deficiency	In children: slow development, mental dullness, retardation, poor bone development In adults: brittle bones, falling/greying hair, fading memory, late periods, infertility, low sperm count and failure to develop normally

Jing has two sources. The most important is our parents and can be described as our constitution. The other source is gained throughout life and is the daily creation of energy from food, drink and the air we breathe. This created energy helps to support the constitutionally based Jing. Together they constitute our Jing.

Jing might be compared to a car battery. Some batteries are better quality than others, and all have a natural lifetime. If we don't overuse the battery by leaving the lights on and driving only at night, then it will last a normal time. Over-using the battery will cause it to run out more quickly. Abusing ourselves by stress, strain, overwork, poor food and irregular eating will deplete our Jing and shorten our life.

Jing controls our ability to reproduce and to develop normally. The development associated with Jing is longer term – thought of as seven-year cycles for women and eight for men. These cycles are spoken of in the language of images rather than biochemistry. Reference is made to: growth in hair, teeth, puberty; the onset of menstruation; the beginning of sexual arousal; fertility; changes in complexion; the falling of hair; the decay of teeth, menopause; infertility; decrease in sexual fluids; drying up of other fluids; and finally the decreasing ability of the brain to function. Underlying our life cycle from birth to death is the notion of Jing.

Westerners are quick to ask, 'Can we increase our Jing?' The Chinese believed that Jing could be improved by herbs and exercises such as Qi Gong. Tai Ji and meditation also help to preserve the Jing. But the main emphasis when dealing with Jing deficiencies is caring for the post-birth Jing – good food, appropriate exercise, adequate rest and a regular life – and adapting our lifestyle to the level of our inherited constitutional strength.

'Adapting our lifestyle' means that we stop doing what wears us out and depletes our energy. This means, on a daily basis, getting sufficient rest, tender loving care, and relaxation. It is noticeable in the West that, in spite of our material prosperity, more people tend to live stressed and overworked lives. We rarely reinvest our energy; instead we spend our Qi wildly and use our energy credit card liberally. This results in an earlier depletion of Jing and an increasing number of chronic, degenerative diseases.

So the better question is, 'How do we best preserve Jing?' Your herbalist may, after careful consideration, give you some advice as to how to change your lifestyle to better preserve your Jing.

With respect to the sexes, Chinese medicine says that men are more prone to Jing Deficiency than women. This is not the Jing Deficiency that occurs before birth, but that which occurs as life proceeds. The reason for this is that, during sex, men lose sperm and women lose nothing of comparable value. Sperm is thought to be the clearest physical manifestation of Jing. Therefore *excessive* sexual activity by a man gradually leads to earlier greying of the hair, sore knees, weak legs, decay of teeth and decline of brain function – all symptoms associated with decreasing Jing. This controversial view creates much discussion in the West – especially about the meaning of 'excessive' – but it is a view that the Chinese take seriously.

Closely related to Jing is the next Substance, Blood.

Blood

'Blood' is both similar and different to our Western understanding. The Chinese do think of Blood as the red fluid which flows through our arteries and veins. Its functions, however, are described differently from those in a Western medical text. Blood is said, simply, to nourish, to moisten and to house the Shen. So what are the imbalances of Blood and how would we recognise them by their symptoms?

Blood imbalance	Typical signs and symptoms
Blood Deficiency	Pale dull face, pale lips, light-headedness, pins and needles, numbness, tremors, blurred vision, poor memory, insomnia, dryness; thin pulse, pale, dry tongue
Blood Stagnation	Severe, fixed, boring, stabbing pain; masses which do not move, purple nails and lips, dark complexion, bleeding with dark blood, menstrual clots; wiry or choppy pulse, purple tongue
Heat in the Blood	Feeling very hot; red and raised skin rashes; heavy bleeding not from trauma

Blood Deficiency and Blood Stagnation are the commonly occurring imbalances. Blood Deficiency, because the Blood is said to house the Shen, easily leads to Shen Disturbance which was described above. Indeed, the insomnia listed under Blood Deficiency could also be said to be a Shen Deficiency symptom. Blood and Shen overlap.

Blood Deficiency occurs frequently in the West. It often occurs from blood loss, for example during childbirth, but more frequently occurs as the result of poor diet, heavy periods or chronic worry and emotional stress. It is not the same as anaemia although patients who are anaemic, based on a Western blood test, can also be Blood Deficient according to Chinese medicine.

Women are more prone to Blood Deficiency than men, just as men are more prone to Jing Deficiency. The reason is their monthly loss of blood. Hence, women suffer more frequently from the pale dull complexion, the light-headedness, cramping of muscles, pins and needles, and the Shen Disturbance which arises when the Blood is deficient and the Shen is not rooted. This may explain our belief that women are more 'emotional' than men.

Blood Stagnation is literally a sluggishness or 'stickiness' of the Blood. One of the key symptoms is pain and the pain is different from the coming and going of Qi Stagnation pain referred to above. This pain is more fixed in location, more stabbing in quality and more continuous. The clotting of menstrual blood and the clotting of blood in a coronary artery are both example of Blood Stagnation. The other typical symptom of Blood Stagnation is fixed lumps or tumours, whether they are painful or not. Fibroids, endometriosis and many cancers are described in Chinese medicine as Blood Stagnation.

Often, because the Qi and Blood are said to move together, Blood Stagnation is a development from Qi Stagnation, and the symptoms are correspondingly more severe.

We can now look at the last Substance, Body Fluids.

Body Fluids

Body Fluids are simply the fluids of the body other than the Blood. Although they are considered Substances, they are thought to be less refined and less essential than Qi, Shen or Blood. They include perspiration, saliva, gastric juices and the synovial fluid of a joint.

The Chinese divide them into two categories, the thinner called 'Jin' and the thicker called 'Ye'. The thinner have the function of moistening and to some extent, like Blood, nourishing. They move with the Protective Qi and manifest as tears, mucus, perspiration and saliva. The thicker move with the Qi and moisten the orifices of sense Organs and moisten joints, spine and brain.

The imbalances of Body Fluids are as follows.

Body Fluid imbalance	Typical signs and symptoms
Deficiency	Dryness of lips, skin, hair, mucus membranes
Accumulation	Any excess of fluids, oedema

We have now looked at the basic Substances and seen how the Substance imbalances are used to classify symptoms and signs. The existence of the resulting basic patterns is important to the herbalist. In the first place, she will use these basic patterns to point to which herbal prescriptions should be used for the patient. A patient who is Qi Deficient will need a prescription which 'tonifies the Qi'; a patient who is Blood Deficient will need a prescription which 'nourishes the Blood'. In the second place, she will further refine these patterns by 'adding in' the relevant Organ. Not only will someone be Blood Deficient, but they may be either Heart Blood Deficient (the example at the beginning of the chapter) or Liver Blood Deficient or both.

So the patterns which derive from Substance imbalances are made more exact by bringing in the relevant Organ. We will now turn to the Organs and their functions to show how they further refine the patterns.

Organs

If the Substances are the material of life, the Organs are the factories which create, store and distribute the Substances. So the most important functions of the Organs are described in relation to Substances. For example, the Spleen and Lungs create Qi. The Heart stores the Shen and the Liver stores the Blood. The Spleen and Lungs help distribute Qi and Body Fluids. Thus, the weakness or strength of an Organ will in turn affect a Substance which in turn will produce various symptoms. We will now examine the five main Organs – the Heart, Spleen, Lungs, Kidney and Liver – and how they each affect the Substances.

It is useful here to remember that the Chinese and Western view of an Organ, although similar, are different. The Chinese Organ is a function first and piece of flesh second. The Chinese speak about what the Organ does and specifically how it affects the Substances. So I will refer to the 'Heart', not the heart – just to keep this distinction clear.

Heart

The Heart has two main functions. The first is that it 'governs the Blood and the Blood vessels'. So the Heart is responsible for the movement of blood and for the Chinese the heart, the blood and the blood vessels are all part of one system. Problems to do with the blood or circulation will often be part of a pattern which involves the Heart.

The second function is that the Heart stores the Shen. The Shen is our Mind or Spirit and governs the functions of thinking, sleeping, consciousness and memory. So when these functions are out of sorts, this is often a result of the Heart not storing the Shen.

Insomnia is an example. The Chinese say that during the day it is natural for the Mind to be directed outwards. But in the evening, when it is time to sleep, the Mind naturally returns inside to the Heart Blood. 'Heart Blood' is a phrase meaning the aspect of the Blood under control of the Heart. If the Heart Blood is deficient, then the Shen will not find its 'bed' comfortable and as a result sleep will be difficult. To cure the insomnia, we need to 'nourish the Heart Blood'.

A typical symptom of the heart is 'palpitations'. Having palpitations means that on occasions a person will feel their heart beat, and not just when they have been exercising. Palpitations as a symptom is common to many of the heart patterns.

Lungs

As the Heart is related to the Substance Blood, the Lungs are related to Qi. The Lungs are said to 'govern Qi and respiration'. This means that the state of our energy or Qi depends on the functioning of our Lungs. Lungs are said to 'descend the Qi' and this can be understood, in part, as inhalation. When this function is good, breathing can be deep, smooth and regular. When it is poor, there can be various symptoms such as a weak voice, not wanting to speak, coughs, asthma and other difficulties of breathing.

We said above that 'protection' was one of the functions of Qi. This job is done by the Lungs. The Lungs 'disperse' the Protective Qi between the skin and muscles. This Protective Qi enables us to open and close our pores and thereby control sweating. It also enables us to ward off excess climatic conditions, which for the Chinese are the 'causes' of many infections, colds and flus. Thus someone prone to colds may benefit from herbs which strengthen the Lungs.

Curiously, as well as protecting in this way, the Lungs are called the 'uppermost' Organ which means that they are particularly vulnerable to the external climate. If the weather is cold and damp, then cold and damp air is breathed directly into the Lungs themselves. This understanding of the Lungs as the 'uppermost' Organ leads the Chinese to practise great care when the weather is inclement. It is not unusual in December in Beijing to see a group of cyclists all wearing cotton masks over their mouths to moderate the harshness of the weather.

Liver

The Liver has two main functions. The first is to 'ensure the smooth flow of Qi'. To Westerners this is a curious notion – that the job of one Organ is to maintain regularity and smoothness throughout the energy of the whole body. But when the Liver is not right, many irregularities appear. These include: a woman never knowing when her period will come, breathing problems which come and go with no reason; digestion which is fine for a few days and then terrible for a few days; bowels moving from diarrhoea to constipation and back; and mood swings (often involving anger or depression) which seem out of control and interfere with the smooth flow of life. A dysfunction of the Liver can cause almost any irregularity.

As a pattern, this is called 'Liver Qi Stagnation'. Significantly, when the Liver disturbs the regularity of another Organ, for example the Lungs, and causes tightness of the chest and difficulty in breathing, there may be nothing wrong with the Lungs themselves. In spite of the Lungs' symptoms, treatment of the Lungs themselves will make no difference. What is needed is treatment of the Liver – called 'smoothing the irregular Liver Qi'. Hence the importance of the herbalist determining the correct Organ and thus the correct pattern.

The other function of the Liver is to store the Blood. The Chinese say that when a person moves, the Blood flows through the body; when a person rests, the Blood returns to the Liver. So this 'storing' function involves both the 'regulation' of the Blood, (the blood getting to the right places at the right time), and the sufficiency of the Blood. Typical symptoms which result from the Liver not storing properly are dryness and tiredness of the eyes, injuries and stiffness of tendons, light-headedness upon standing, cramps, pins and needles, and excessive or insufficient menstrual flows.

Spleen / Pancreas

The main function of the Spleen is to create Qi via its control over the digestive system. In this respect, the Spleen is said to 'transform' and 'transport'. 'Transforming' refers to the process whereby food and drink are converted into energy. This process involves movement, for example of the material through the digestive system and hence the 'transporting' as well as the 'transforming'.

When the transforming function is not strong, then the production of Qi or energy is poor and typically there will be tiredness and digestive symptoms such as poor appetite, loose stools (sometimes with undigested food) and a heavy feeling after eating. Because of this function, the Spleen is said to be a source of post-birth energy, whereas the Kidney, because it stores the Jing, is said to be the source of pre-birth energy.

The Spleen has two other functions which relate to the Substances. The first is that it carries out the 'moving upwards of Qi'. This means that any excessive downward movement, such as diarrhoea, a prolapse, or simply a downward bearing sensation in the abdomen comes from a Spleen weakness. In this context, the Spleen also take the clear, bright energy to the head and thus creates a clear mind. A fuzzy, unclear mind often indicates a poor Spleen function.

The second function is 'to hold the Blood in the Blood vessels'. This means that some sorts of bleeding, particularly those where the blood leaks slowly, may be due to a Spleen weakness. Bleeding from the uterus outside the period is often due to the Spleen. Small red spots on the skin formed by leakage of Blood from the Blood vessels are a minor example.

Kidneys

The Kidney stores the Jing which governs the long-term cycles of growth, development and reproduction. So any of the Jing Deficiency symptoms discussed above – such as infertility, premature aging, impotence or retarded growth – would be treated by herbs which affect the Kidneys.

The Kidneys also produce 'marrow', which has not been mentioned yet, but is a material that is related to Jing. The Chinese said that 'marrow' is common to bones, bone marrow, the spinal cord and brain. A deficiency of the Kidneys can produce a weakness of the bones (as in the osteoporosis at menopause), problems of the spine and a dullness of mind.

The Kidneys are also said to be the 'root of life'. This means that, to some degree, all other Organs are dependent upon the Kidneys for their Yin or Yang energy. The Yang energy, you may remember, is the warming, moving energy; the Yin energy is the nourishing, cooling energy. Although the Organs affect each other, the Spleen Yang energy, for example, depends more on the Kidney Yang than vice versa. As a result, many Chinese doctors will always carefully consider – through examination of the pulse and tongue – whether the Kidneys are functioning well. If not, even if the problems seem to be coming from another Organ, the herbalist will include in the prescription some herbs to strengthen the Kidneys.

So we can see how a specific Organ is more closely related to one Substance than another, and how the symptoms arising from the weakness of an Organ are often explained via the related Substance pathology. We can summarise the connection between Organs and Substances in the following table.

Organ	Substances affected
Heart	Blood, Shen
Lungs	Qi, Body Fluids
Liver	Qi, Blood
Spleen	Qi, Body Fluids
Kidney	Jing, Qi, Body Fluids

We need to consider one more piece of theory to understand all the terms used in the label for a pattern – the Pathogenic Factors or the 'Evil External Influences'.

Evil External Influences

The ancient Chinese understood that a harsh climate causes illness. Under normal circumstances, a person with good Protective Qi can withstand the weather and retain good health. But when the weather is excessive or the person's Protective Qi is weak, the climate, so to speak, 'gets in' and creates illness. For the ancient Chinese, these climates were Wind, Cold, Damp, Fire, Summer Heat and Dryness. They remain a common explanation of how we become ill.

Observation led to a further use of this notion. Climates, as well as being causes of disease, are also used to label certain patterns of signs and symptoms. This means that words like 'Wind' and 'Cold' were not just used as descriptions of the weather and 'causes' of illness; they were also used to describe the patterns of disharmony affecting a person. For example, a person with a common cold may have the pattern 'Wind and Cold invading the Lungs'. These patterns, like others, are also described through signs and symptoms.

So climates are a cause of illness and the language of climates is used in the description of patterns. A climate, when 'stuck in the inside', is called a Pathogenic Factor. In Chinese medicine, this means that it needs to be cleared or expelled. Let us see how this works out in practise.

Wind

Wind as a cause often works together with one of the other Evil Influences. For example, Wind and Cold often combine. One of the ways that Wind and Cold combine and Wind helps to cause disease is currently expressed in our notion of the 'chill factor'. Only in the past few years have weather reports included the 'chill factor'. Chill factor simply means that if it is 5°C outside, it will feel a lot colder if there is a strong wind. For this reason, the Chinese said that 'Wind is the spearhead of disease' and causes Cold to penetrate.

Wind as a pattern of disharmony is similar to wind in nature. We often observe wind as it moves the branches of a tree. The wind blows intermittently, arises quickly, moves upward and outward, and makes things shake and sway. Such are the symptoms associated with Wind. Wind symptoms are ones that come on quickly and move around: a pain that come on overnight and is in one joint one day, and another the next day. Wind symptoms often affect the top part of the body or the 'uppermost Organ', the Lungs. Wind often affects the skin, and causes itching which comes and goes. 'Wind' is the explanation or description of many tics, tremors and convulsions.

Cold

Cold is familiar to most of us as a cause of disease. In ancient Northern China, there were many months of freezing weather without central heating and without thermal underwear. The Chinese character for Cold was a picture which included a shelter, a man and straw. We cannot be certain, but the picture conjured up is a man who is buried in straw to keep himself warm.

How is Cold part of the patterns of disharmony? Cold when it penetrates impairs the moving function of Qi. The obstruction created frequently causes pain. Most of us are familiar with, for example, our hands or ears getting so cold that they begin to hurt. Usually, when this happens, we get warm again and the Cold does not get 'stuck' in us. But sometimes, particularly with joints and when the Protective Qi is weak, the Cold enters, gets stuck and over time causes continuing, severe, sharp pain – which feels better when we put heat on it. The curious thing about Cold getting stuck in a joint is that we don't have to feel this kind of Cold as cold – like we do when our ears are suffering from frostbite. This pain will, however, feel temporarily better for the application of heat and will respond to herbs which warm.

Cold frequently gets stuck in joints causing pain, but it can also get stuck in the stomach, intestines or uterus. Too much ice cream in the stomach can result in pain and vomiting which are typical symptoms of 'Cold in the Stomach'. 'Cold in the uterus', which may not be experienced as a feeling of cold, results in obstruction and therefore pain. This pain usually occurs around the time of the period and can be relieved temporarily by a hot water bottle. A more permanent cure can be achieved from herbs which warm the uterus and expel Cold.

Damp

Damp or humidity are climatic conditions where the air contains moisture. The Thames Valley tends to be damp; so does the west coast of Ireland and Baltimore and the Chesapeake Bay area. Working in wet conditions, living in a damp house, wearing wet clothes while sailing, and even washing your hair and letting it dry by itself – all these expose a person to Damp.

What are the patterns of disharmony when Damp has penetrated? Damp is an accumulation of Body Fluids. It is said to obstruct the moving function of Qi, to naturally linger on and to create a feeling of heaviness. Damp can enter different parts of the body, but let us again take a joint as an example.

Damp stuck in a joint results in a pain of fixed location, a feeling of heaviness, soreness and stiffness. The joint may be swollen and it will frequently be somewhat better when it is being moved and get a little worse upon rest. The movement of the joint tends to move the Damp; the lack of movement tends to increase the obstruction and allow the Damp to accumulate.

There are three ways we can become affected by Damp. One is that we are in excessively damp conditions for sufficient time and the external damp penetrates. This process is facilitated when the Protective Qi and the transporting energy of the Spleen are weak. People who live in damp climates are more likely to be affected.

Another way of developing Damp is when the Spleen and Lungs are weak and Body Fluids are not being circulated internally with vigour. The sluggishness of the internal Body Fluids means that some accumulate and this results in Damp. This kind of Damp is often in the digestive system and creates a poor appetite and feeling of fullness after eating only a little.

The last way of developing Damp is through eating what are called 'damp-producing' foods. These are dairy products and greasy foods which are more difficult for the Spleen to transform and which often result in an accumulation of Damp in the digestive system. The symptoms of digestive Damp are a poor appetite ('I already feel full'), a feeling of fullness after eating, and abdominal distension.

So Damp as a pattern of disharmony has different causes. Accordingly, the herbs used to clear Damp will be selected according to how the Damp arose and where it is in the body. The different 'Damps' are an example of how an external climate began to be used as a way of describing internal patterns of disharmony.

Fire

Chinese medicine talks about both Heat and Fire. Heat usually is said to come from the outside. Fire, on the other hand, is internally generated heat. So here we are not talking so much about an external climate, but more an internal climate or pattern of disharmony. In the internal landscape, Heat is more superficial, and Fire more deep.

Heat may manifest in a common cold where the patient feels mainly feverish (only a few chills) and probably has a sore throat. This superficial Wind-Heat might later turn into acute bronchitis where the lungs hurt, the temperature is high, there is much sweating, a great thirst and the patient feels only hot with no chills at all. In this case, the superficial Heat is said to have gone deeper inside the body.

Fire, on the other hand, arises from a deficiency of Body Fluids and from internal Stagnation. Typical symptoms of Fire are a red face, feeling hot, high fevers, boils, loving cool drinks and having a bitter taste in the mouth. Also present might be 'reckless' and profuse bleeding (as in some nosebleeds), and disturbed Shen. Fire, like Wind, tends to move upwards and will easily disturb the Shen, producing dream-disturbed sleep and outbursts of temper. These outbursts will be inappropriate and driven by the excess Fire on the inside.

It is a general clinical rule in Chinese medicine that when there is Fire, it should be cleared first. This means that before using herbs to nourish fluids, it is important first to use herbs that will clear the Fire.

Summer Heat

This Heat is also from the outside. It is not a common cause of disease for most of us. People in hot countries and some people who work, for example, in bakeries or blast furnaces, may have been affected by external Heat. Summer Heat injures Body Fluids and depletes the Qi. Its symptoms include a high fever and heavy sweating.

Dryness

Dryness, like Summer Heat, is not such a common condition or cause of disease. It manifests in a lack of Body Fluids and so has some similarities to Heat. External dryness, which is a lack of moisture in the atmosphere, will interfere with Lungs' function of dispersing and often results in a dry cough and asthmatic conditions. Otherwise, Dryness manifests as dry lips, dry nostrils, dry tongue, dry and cracked skin and constipation with dry stools.

This a brief description of the Evil External Influences. They are both external climatic causes and also patterns of disharmony. As far as patterns go, there is one more term to consider as it also ranks as a Pathogenic Factor alongside Wind, Damp, Cold and the others. This other Substance is called Phlegm.

Phlegm

The 'Phlegm' of Chinese medicine does include our ordinary notion of Phlegm – the Phlegm which comes from our lungs when we cough it up. To the Chinese it means more. At the risk of over-simplifying, Phlegm is any sticky material which has accumulated in the body and is blocking the flow of Qi and Blood. It is thicker than Damp, which does the same, and it tends to produce more severe symptoms. In the head it can cause vertigo or severe dizziness. In the throat it can produce a restricted feeling and difficulty in swallowing. In the chest, tightness, pressure and pain. In the abdomen, masses or lumps, benign or malignant. In the limbs, numbness and insensitivity. In the joints of the hands and feet, knobbly lumps.

Phlegm is created internally when the Spleen is not transforming and moving properly. In this respect it is like Damp. You would not be far wrong if you think of it as Damp which has condensed and got thicker.

So now we have a wider description of the dirt which gets in the machine. The dirt is the Pathogenic Factors which need to be cleared or expelled.

Putting it all together

Let us return to your visit to the herbalist. You are with the herbalist who is getting to know you. You mention your complaints. She takes your pulse and looks at your tongue. She asks questions, listens to you, and goes inside her head to consult the 'patterns'. She sifts, refines and puts the pieces together. All she is doing is looking for patterns. The vocabulary of the patterns are Organs, Substances and Pathogenic Factors. Some Organs and Substances will require strengthening and some Pathogenic Factors will require clearing.

The above is theory. Let us now look at some patients and observe the patterns of disharmony in action.

4

Patients' Stories

Who goes for Chinese herbs? And, what do Chinese herbs help?

Who goes for Chinese herbs?

There has been no survey of who visits a Chinese herbalist. Based on my own experience and from what I know of colleagues, there are a few generalisations. One is that the range of people is very wide – all ages, all walks of life and all sorts of complaints. On the other hand, there are probably slightly more women than men and more people in the age range 35 to 50. The only other significant factor is that fees are charged, which is important when many people, at least in the UK, can visit the doctor for no direct payment. Having said that, many herbalists take the income level of their patients into consideration and under some circumstances reduce fees. Many herbalists will have one day set aside for children and some specialise, for example, in skin problems.

What complaints do herbalists treat?

What do Chinese herbs help? Here is a list of complaints that Chinese herbs help. Anxiety states, arthritis, back pain, circulatory problems, complications following a stroke, depression, fibrositis, high blood pressure, indeterminate aches and pains, infertility, menstrual problems, migraines and other headaches, paralysis and wasting of muscles, rheumatism, sciatica, sequelae of strokes, skin conditions and ulcers.

There are two comments about such a list. The first is that a brief description of a problem is usually not a good basis for a prognosis. Potential patients often telephone and ask if herbs can help their problem. If they have headaches, the answer will almost certainly be 'Yes.' If it is paralysis of a limb then a great deal more information is required. The label of the problem helps the herbalist give some opinion, but the state of the person is also extremely important.

The second comment is that people frequently take herbs even though they do not come under one of the above categories. These may be people who are feeling 'not quite right', but have been told by their doctor there is nothing wrong with them. They come for herbs because the Chinese process of diagnosis does not require that you have a labelled disease. Feeling 'not quite right' is good enough. After all, people who know they are 'not quite right', and yet 'not really sick' are usually people who are in the process of getting ill. Being aware, and seeking help, is an obvious form of intelligence – especially when contrasted with waiting until you are really ill and only then asking for help.

People of that sort often come when they know others who have benefited. They understand enough of the process by hearsay that they anticipate getting help. They usually do.

So let us return to some typical patients. The best way to explain Chinese herbal medicine is to tell some 'patient stories'. These patients have, in general, done well and it is not true that every patient going to a Chinese herbalist has a complete cure. But these ones have had considerable improvement and illustrate the range of complaints that herbal medicine deals with.

Penny

When Penny came for treatment, she was a shy schoolgirl, studying for A levels. Her mother made the appointment and was very distressed for her daughter. Her mother said it was a skin problem which she had had since a baby. When Penny came to the consultation, she seemed awkward and embarrassed. I encountered her sitting in the waiting room, slouched over, covering her face with a book. When she stood up, she was obviously pretty, but her hair and her clothes suggested a 'couldn't care less' attitude. Her face was a pale dull colour. In the treatment room she spoke quickly, looking down:

My mum thinks I should come. Nothing has ever helped me very much. It's getting worse lately and I suppose that's my A levels coming up in three months. I hate it. I just want it to go away. Boy don't like me 'cos of it.

What Penny was talking about was eczema. With the exception of the odd month here or there, Penny had had eczema as far back as she could remember. According to her mother it began when she was four or five months old. The eczema consisted of patches of flaky skin on her hands, elbows, neck and sometimes face. When her hands were bad they would swell up. All the eczema patches would itch and scratching would bring out a yellowish fluid. The recent problem was its spread to her face.

The additional information supporting Penny's diagnosis was as follows.

Penny's appetite was up and down. She rarely ate breakfast, and preferred snacking to eating three regular meals. She ate a lot of cheese, cakes and biscuits – foods high in fat and sugar. She felt tired a lot of the time, preferring when she returned from school to flop in front of the TV. She slept heavily and for over ten hours a night on the weekends. She felt the cold easily and her limbs were cold to the touch. Her digestion was sluggish – she would feel a bit heavy and bloated after eating her evening meal. Her bowel movements were loose.

In addition, Penny's periods were more six-weekly than monthly. Her short-term memory was poor: she frequently forgot her keys and the correct books for school. Any loud sound, or even the telephone ringing, could make her startle on the inside.

Penny's complaint and these other symptoms indicate that Penny is Spleen Yang Deficient, has some Damp and is also Heart Blood Deficient. What does this mean?

The Spleen for the Chinese is equivalent to digestion and transformation and movement in general. When the Spleen is Yang Deficient and does not properly transform and transport, then we often get what is called Damp, which is an accumulation of fluids.

This label, 'Spleen Yang Deficient with Damp', refers to Penny's:

- erratic appetite
- feeling of heaviness after eating a large meal
- loose bowels
- tiredness and heavy sleeping
- general feeling of the body being sluggish
- 'couldn't care less' mental attitude
- yellowish fluid which oozed from her eczema
- empty and slippery pulse
- swollen tongue.

Eating heavy and greasy food does not help this problem. Most greasy food is 'Damp-forming', implying that if you eat too much of this type of food, even if your Spleen is strong, you will accumulate 'Damp'. When you are Damp you are more likely to feel tired and heavy limbed.

Penny was also 'Heart Blood Deficient'. Penny's signs of this pattern were:

- poor short-term memory
- being easily startled
- poor concentration
- a pale dull-looking face.

This pattern comes from various causes. The three main ones are loss of blood, poor diet and both worry and anxiety. When women give birth and lose a lot of blood, they will temporarily become 'Heart Blood Deficient' and as a result suffer from many mental symptoms, including depression. In Penny's case, the Heart Blood Deficiency probably came more from her poor digestion and poor diet and was made worse by her feeling anxious. Green vegetables 'nourish the Blood' and Penny only rarely ate vegetables. In Penny's case, the symptoms were not severe, but overall the poor short-term memory, poor concentration and 'Damp'-type tiredness were making her less able to cope.

Penny was given herbs to clear Damp, strengthen her Spleen and nourish her Blood. At first she was given a prescription consisting of dried herbs which she had to 'decoct'. Decocting is putting the herbs in water, bringing the water to the boil and then simmering for 20 minutes. The resulting decoction is drunk and one bag provides enough for two days.

Penny was seen again when she finished the first ten bags. The eczema was clear from her face, for which she was delighted, but it was still present on the neck, hands and elbows although to a lesser degree. She looked brighter and said that she was feeling pretty good in herself. Because the eczema fluctuated, it was hard to be sure of any real improvement. The prescription was repeated and another appointment was made for four weeks.

At the next visit Penny's eczema was almost clear, better than she had seen it in the past year. We assumed that the herbs were definitely having an effect. She was feeling well in herself. Studying for her exams was difficult but not a problem, and she said that her appetite was more regular. At this time we discussed what an ideal eating pattern would be and which foods – many of her favourites – were likely to bring the eczema back. She was receptive and it was left to her to make any changes. The herbs were modified.

At Penny's next visit her eczema was almost completely clear and she was feeling well in herself. Her 'couldn't care less' attitude was gone. She was standing straighter, her hair was neat and there was a sparkle in her eye.

Penny then went onto herbal pills. She was no longer 'Heart Blood Deficient' and carried much less 'Damp'. The new formula was for Spleen Deficiency and some Damp. For Penny, pills were much easier to take and the decocted herbs had no advantage.

I spoke to Penny's mother after this and she filled in many gaps. Penny was eating regularly and a much better diet with hardly any Damp-forming foods. Her room had become tidier – I didn't know it wasn't – and she was ready for, and optimistic about, her exams. Her digestion was normal and she no longer felt heavy and bloated after eating.

Her mother said: 'I was worried about her eczema and if I'd known I would have brought her years ago. She is a whole lot better.' I knew she meant this as her next request was whether she could come for herbs herself. No one told me how Penny was getting on with boys, but I assumed all was well.

Peter

Peter's wife, who had already been a patient, first made contact. She was interested in alternative medicine, had studied reflexology and had a good understanding of how nutrition affects health. Her problem now, however, was Peter and his tendency to overwork and not get adequate rest.

At the time of the phone call, Peter had ignored an on-and-off cold for five weeks and suddenly developed a high fever. He felt so ill he had gone to bed. He was sweating, felt very hot, was coughing up small amounts of yellow sputum, hurt inside his chest, and was restless and worried about his inability to complete a current project. Peter was not used to being ill. In the past, he had simply worked through any flus or colds. He was unsympathetic to those who took time off to recuperate, but, at that moment, he had had to go to bed.

Living close and knowing his wife, I visited. Peter had first developed a cold after playing football for his team at work. For the month or so before, he had been working particularly hard and reluctantly admitted that he was very tired.

Herbalists would describe the common cold as an 'invasion of Wind-Cold or Wind-Heat', depending upon the pattern of symptoms and in particular the degree of 'Cold' signs as opposed to 'Heat' signs. Prior to going to bed, Peter had developed more 'Wind-Heat' signs. He was still feeling nervous about going out in the cold, but more feeling hot and occasionally sweating. His throat was sore and his nose was running with yellow mucus.

There are herbal remedies to take at this moment, but adequate rest is an essential part of getting better. The

Chinese talk of the Wind and Heat invading the body and the 'Upright Qi', or your background level of good energy, doing battle with the Wind and Heat. One good way to support your 'Upright Qi' is to get adequate rest regularly. Peter had not rested.

Because he didn't rest, Peter's 'Wind-Heat', in the Chinese description, went deeper, overcame the 'upright Qi' and became interior rather than exterior 'Heat'. The label for his current condition was 'Heat in the Lung'. The signs and symptoms are:

- high fever
- feeling hot
- coughing with yellow sputum
- sweating
- a rapid and full pulse
- a red tongue body with a yellow coating.

At this point the Chinese principle of treatment is to 'clear the Heat from the Lung' and a formula with five herbs in it was used. This particular combination of herbs is not available in a pill, and dry herbs which the patient boils up, or 'decocts', have a stronger, more immediate effect.

What were Peter's other options? One was simply to remain in bed, rest and hope that he got better. This was not a good option in the view of Chinese medicine. As his 'Upright Qi' was weak, the fever which was varying from 103–104°F would probably have remained for several days and that could have left him recovered, but not quite right. 'Recovered, but not quite right' applies when people get over an illness, but say later that they have never been quite right ever since the illness. Chinese medicine describes this as a Pathogenic Factor getting stuck in the system. ME or post-viral syndrome is one common example.

Peter's Western diagnosis would have been acute bronchitis and his other option was to take antibiotics. The Chinese view on antibiotics is mixed and antibiotics are definitely used in China. It is clear that antibiotics would be better than simply resting. The view of traditional Chinese medicine is that the risk with antibiotics is that they stop the infection, but they do not always result in a natural clearing of the Heat and Phlegm accompanying the infection. The consequence again is that the patient can be 'recovered, but not quite right'.

Peter, partly under-influence of his wife, opted for the herbs. I explained at this point that we needed to approach the illness in stages, warning Peter that he was not to return to full speed just because he felt a little better. My concern was to clear the Heat and then to give him herbs which would strengthen his resistance. My worry was that as soon as he felt better, he would forget about herbs and resume his rigorous life.

Over five days, taking the herbs two to three times each day, Peter gradually improved. He no longer had any of the signs and symptoms of 'Lung Heat', but he did feel weak and still had a slight, non-productive cough. He and his wife had talked about his passion for work and its effect on him and the family. When he next visited the clinic he showed some signs that his Yin energy, the nourishing, cooling and wetter energy, had been damaged. His signs and symptoms were:

- mild, unproductive cough

- a tongue body which was red, without much coat and with a few horizontal cracks in the Lung area

- a dry mouth and throat

- feeling slightly warmer in the afternoon although the temperature was normal

- a floating and slightly rapid pulse.

Peter was then given a formula to 'strengthen his Lung Yin' and after ten days he felt much stronger, and the above signs and symptoms had disappeared. He felt well enough that he was becoming anxious to go back to work. He was told that he should do so, but with a shorter day for at least a week and a commitment not to bring work home.

This was a difficult moment, but being reminded of the day he felt very ill and how it had all occurred, he agreed. He continued to take another formula in pill form which was designed to strengthen both his 'Lung Qi' and his Protective Qi. If you remember from Chapter 3, the Protective Qi is part of the Lungs' energy and is sometimes called the 'defensive' energy. Six months later he was living a better lifestyle and coming in for three-monthly checks.

There is an obvious lesson here. Looking after oneself is important. In this case, adequate rest and relaxation is the issue. In our Western culture many of us have a credit card attitude to our energy. That is, we spend until we are empty and then, using credit, we spend a little more. We deplete our Jing and thereby lower our immune responses. Peter's illness is only one of many that this attitude encourages.

Gerry

Gerry was ten when he first came for herbs. His headmaster had just stopped him attending PE classes and told his parents to take him to a doctor and get an inhaler. The reason was that during PE, especially cross-country running, Gerry would become breathless and take 30 minutes to an hour to recover.

Gerry was pear-shaped and wore T-shirts emblazoned with pop group logos. He played the guitar and his preference for 'casual' dress and his general slowness and untidiness upset his mother. She wanted the best for him and the conflict between her and his ideas (it was her idea he take herbs) resulted in Gerry being initially withdrawn and difficult to take information from. I asked his mum to wait outside while Gerry and I talked.

If it had not been for the T-shirt, I would not have known where to start. I asked Gerry about his favourite groups and we only gradually got back to talking about him.

Cold and any strenuous activity, like playing football, made Gerry breathless. It had got worse over the last three years. Gerry's solution was to stay inside and play the guitar. The teachers sent him outside to run. In the winter time he frequently caught colds and would cough up large amounts of white sputum. The breathlessness would be worse when he had a cold, but, on exertion, could occur at any time.

Various signs pointed to Gerry's Kidneys. The facial colour associated with the Kidneys is black. Gerry had this colour under his eyes and he also had one other important Kidney sign. When the Lungs are energetically weak, breathlessness is experienced more on breathing out. With the Kidneys, it is breathing in. Gerry easily made this distinction and said his problem was breathing in.

Saying that it was the Kidneys rather than the Lungs often makes Chinese medicine difficult for Westerners. The breathlessness is still manifesting in the physical lungs. What the Chinese theory is saying is that a change will occur if we strengthen the energy of the Kidneys, rather than the Lungs.

What else was significant? Gerry slouched which inhibits good breathing and ultimately weakens the lungs. He adored pizzas and generally preferred Burger King to McDonald's, although it was close. His diet, which contained many

'Phlegm-forming' foods, clearly contributed to his wheezing. Phlegm-forming foods and a weakened underlying energy make the normal transformation of food less successful with the result that more 'Phlegm' accumulates in the body.

The diagnosis was that his Kidney energy, especially his Kidney Yang energy, was weak and that he frequently had 'Damp and Phlegm obstructing his Lungs'.

Gerry was given herbal pills. He was given one pill to warm and strengthen his underlying Kidney energy and another to take whenever he had accumulated Phlegm in his lungs.

Gerry's improvement was gradual over the winter. I saw him seven times over five months from October to the end of February. He was then able to play a game of football without any breathlessness. He had had only three colds which was exceptional compared to the winter before. His slouch and general withdrawal was gone. His passion for music and the guitar, if anything, had increased and, surprising to him, his mother was supporting him by paying for lessons with a teacher outside school. His mother spoke to me about him in a very different tone.

People, when getting better, change in many ways and it is one of the herbalist's satisfactions to notice these. I first saw Gerry five years ago and have seen him at least twice a year since that time. He has taken herbs on and off over the five years, although more off than on. He looks well now. He has no problems with breathing, he stands upright and he has a healthy passion for life. Even his mother is proud of his guitar playing.

What can we learn from Gerry? One thing is that the herbalist will not always focus on the Organ which appears to be the problem. Strengthening Gerry's Lungs would not have made him better. Hence the importance of the correct diagnosis. Another lesson is that getting stronger often produces a variety of changes in the person and even in the folks around them. It often is a small difference in vital energy that stops a vicious downward spiral and changes it into a beneficent, upward spiral. Herbs can sometimes start that process off. The other thing to learn is the value of early treatment. It is not that treatment later in life is wasted. But the value of a good change at Gerry's age is significant. Not going through puberty labelled 'asthmatic' allows Gerry to be more himself.

Carol

Carol announced her name and complaint in a loud and clipped voice over the telephone. In two minutes, she had asked multiple questions about time, money, how to take the herbs, how long it would take, and so on. I might have been talking to an engineer about the specification for a machine. She explained that she had been a computer programmer, but was just finishing her accountancy exams and about to take on a new and important job.

Carol was 29, and suffering from period pains. She described the pain as 'horrendous' and the worst thing she had ever experienced. Her cycle was irregular – from 23 to 34 days. The pains were stabbing, went right through her and made her incapable for three days a month. Although she had had some form of pain ever since her first period, they were generally worse when she was stressed and had been much worse in the past six months. The pains started two days before the period and continued for two days into the period. She had tried a variety of pain killers, but none had helped significantly.

Carol had a short but successful career in computer programming and her study of accountancy was the stepping stone to a promising job which required both skills. She had the job, subject to her passing the accountancy exams. But she didn't believe she could keep the job if she continued to have three days a month suffering from incapacitating pain. Although she had heard from a friend that Chinese herbs tasted awful, she said she would try anything.

You may remember in Chapter 3 where we compared the pain from Qi Stagnation and Blood Stagnation. Blood is more solid than Qi, and Blood Stagnation pain is more severe – often described as stabbing – and often fixed in one place, and continuous. Carol had a mixture of both types of pain and her diagnosis was 'Qi and Blood Stagnation in the Uterus'. The other signs and symptoms which supported this were: a tongue body which was purple, large clots in the menstrual blood which she remembers from her teens, a slightly green colour around her eyes and mouth, a pulse which felt like a stretched wire, and eight days of pre-menstrual tension characterised by a great deal of edginess and explosive outbursts of anger. Concerning the outbursts, she said, 'They are *not* ladylike and I need to keep them under control.'

The main Organ involved was the Liver with its job of making the Qi flow smoothly. Stagnation results when this Organ is impaired. You may also remember that anger is the emotion associated with the Liver. Carol remembered many moments as a child when she had raged at her strict father who was uncompromising and treated her even more severely the more she rebelled.

The treatment for Carol was herbs to 'smooth' the Liver and specifically to 'move Qi and Blood' in the uterus. The formula used was a modification of one first written down in around 200 AD.

Carol was only four days from a period and this one was like the others. By the next, however, she had taken herbs for a full month and through the premenstrual time. This period was bearable and she said: 'A few stabbing pains the day before, but generally much, much better. Any of my friends would die if they had a period like that, but for me, much, much better.' Carol's pulses were less wiry even though we were again in the pre-period phase.

It was five months before Carol was virtually free of both premenstrual tension and the pain before and during her period. She was then given a prescription, which smoothed the Liver Qi, to be taken only in the latter half of her cycle. A year later her anger was well under control, she was successful in her new job and coming every three months for check-ups. She became, as she described it, much less 'gung ho', was successful in her new work and leading a gentler lifestyle. Her speech was softer and much slower.

One of the interesting lessons here is how the patient's complaint is often expressed in so many other ways – once you know the underlying principles of Chinese medicine. Carol's 'gung ho' behaviour and aggressive approach to life was an expression of Stagnant Liver Qi. Her mind quite rightly focused on the pain. However, in many cases of successful treatment, the herbs have an impact, not just on the symptoms, but on the whole person.

Graham

Graham is a self-taught electrician. As a child he repaired his mother's vacuum cleaner and became what he called 'the repairman of the house'. In business, he regards himself as a secret Robin Hood, charging full prices to those who can afford them and less to those who cannot.

When he rang up, he had been so exhausted that he had only worked two days a week for the last three months. His income was down and, because of his tiredness, as he put it, 'My two kids have given up on me.' In spite of this, during the telephone conversation, he kept asking whether

I thought he really needed treatment. He seemed reluctant to go for help.

Specifically, Graham felt very tired. On his worst days, he would walk upstairs and have to sit down for 20 minutes. His limbs felt heavy and achy. His abdomen felt full and his head fuzzy. He would sleep ten hours a night and still find it hard to wake up. His appetite was erratic. For two days he would eat very little and then binge on sweets and microwaved pizzas. He would have diarrhoea three to five times a day, often waking to go at 5 to 6 a.m. He said, 'It's as if my body and my mind are bogged down in sticky toffee.'

Graham's pulse was slippery and his pale tongue had a thickish white coating.

We mentioned Graham's diagnosis in Chapter 1: a weak Spleen and Kidney with accumulated Damp leading to lethargy and diarrhoea. Part of the Damp is in the muscles; part is in the digestive system. If you remember from Chapter 3, the Spleen is responsible for transforming food and drink into energy. A weak Spleen means low energy. It also means that fluids are not thoroughly transformed and accumulate, leading to heaviness, tiredness and diarrhoea.

Graham had been told that he had ME or post-viral syndrome. Typically, the tiredness had come on after a bout of flu where he felt very achy and was stuffed up with mucus and Phlegm. ME is spoken of as a new disease, but the principles governing the typical ME symptoms have always been clear in Chinese medicine. There is frequently a mixture of Damp and Heat in the muscles with a weak Spleen and weak Kidneys. Both Chinese herbs and acupuncture have a good success record with ME.

Graham had almost no Heat. Damp was the primary pathogen. The treatment principles, which arise out of the diagnosis, are to strengthen the Spleen and Kidneys and to clear Damp.

With someone like Graham, the herbalist's question is which gets the priority, strengthening the weak Organs or clearing the Damp? This is a clinical judgement based on the relative fullness and emptiness – the fullness being the Damp and the emptiness being the Spleen and Kidney. Think of a blocked drain. When a drain is thoroughly blocked, it is necessary first to clear rather than push more water through.

In Graham's case, the priority was placed on the Damp clearing action. He was given ten bags of herbs. Each bag is decocted twice and the ten bags last 20 days. Decocting means covering the herbs with water in a saucepan, bringing the water to a boil, and then simmering for 20 to 30 minutes.

Graham was also asked to change his diet. He was asked to eat consistently, preferably earlier in the day. He was also asked to almost exclude foods which encourage the body to form Damp. These are dairy products and any food containing grease. For Graham this meant not eating the pizzas, cheese and chips he liked so much.

Graham returned after taking the first herbs. He had changed his eating pattern and diet. His energy was considerably better. He had worked four days in each of the last two weeks and two mornings he had woken feeling 'almost normal'. The diarrhoea was somewhat improved. Based on his pulse and tongue he was asked to repeat the same prescription for another 20 days.

Graham visited another six times, roughly at three-weekly intervals. The second time he returned he was working almost full time, but still feeling very tired by late afternoon. For at least the first part of the day his muscles did not ache and he was much more able to concentrate. His diarrhoea was much better. His prescription was modified to be more strengthening and less clearing. On subsequent visits his prescriptions were made more strengthening until, on the last visit, he was given a prepared remedy which he ordered from the herbal dispensary. This final remedy strengthens the Spleen and to a small degree clears Damp. Graham took this for four weeks. I saw him six months later in his role as an electrician. He looked well and said that, except for a couple of bad days, he was fine.

Graham's case raises the question of when to stop having herbs. This is usually a matter of discussion between the patient and practitioner. The patient is the final judge. It is his or her standards of well-being and assessment of the progress to date that count.

What the herbalist can contribute is whether the patient is stopping too soon. There is a moment when the symptoms are gone, but the patient could still be stronger, thereby creating some reserves. For the herbalist, the pulse and tongue are important indicators. There may also be 'symptoms' or signs observed by the herbalist which he knows could be improved. These can be raised and discussed. But the choice is the patient's.

Brenda

Brenda was a 52-year-old yoga teacher. Her hair was grey and had been so for 20 years. Yoga took her all over the country and abroad, teaching both students and teachers. Her posture was very upright and her eyes were intense. She practised at least two hours every day and on many days taught another five to six hours. She had definitely worked hard at her yoga.

How she began yoga was interesting. When young she was always poorly. At 18 she said she was 'taken by a mysterious illness'. She remembers little now except that she was frail and spent a couple of months in bed. Her aunt, who was a yoga teacher, visited her twice a week and taught her some breathing techniques. She attributes her recovery to her aunt and the breathing. She studied with her aunt and early on became a teacher This whole experience, and her understanding of yoga, had led her to be very careful with her health. Before her 'mysterious illness', she had started her periods at 16 and they occurred only irregularly, having six or seven in a year.

Her reason for coming was 'menopause and hot flushes'. For the past three months, she was having five to six flushes a day and these could involve severe feelings of heat and discomfort. Teaching yoga was difficult, as she said, 'with smoke coming out of my ears'.

Brenda's diagnosis was a Blood and Kidney Yin Deficiency. The Yin energy is the nourishing, cooling energy. When this diminishes, which is natural at Brenda's age, the lack of cooling energy allows Heat to flare upwards. The remedy is to use herbs which clear the Heat and nourish the Yin. In Brenda's case, we also nourished Blood.

Brenda was clear of the hot flushes in five weeks. She also noticed that she felt calmer. She asked if it were possible that her muscles would be stretching more easily. I explained how the Blood nourishes the tendons and that she should be stretching better and feeling less aches. As a result of this conversation, Brenda asked for more herbs. We agreed to monitor the effect of these by her feeling of calmness and the feeling of comfort in her body when doing yoga.

Brenda's initial problem is a common one. Chinese herbal medicine has responded to this complaint for over two thousand years and has several formulae designed to clear Heat and nourish the Yin.

Roger

Roger was a farmer. He came for herbs because his five-year-old daughter had had asthma, and herbs had helped her.

Roger had inherited the farm from his father and before that had worked on the farm. He worked long hours, both labouring and managing. His farm was prospering, but he never employed anyone to take over some of the physical work because he preferred working to socialising. He was close to his wife and two children, but otherwise, as he put it, 'happy with his own company'.

His problem was back pain. Even in the summer it was sore and stiff. When lifting bales of hay he frequently had to rest. In the winter the pain became severe and the background ache remained. The mornings were bad until he had a long hot shower. He would be fine for a while, but the more he lifted and the colder it was, the worse the pain became. In addition to the aches and pains, Roger felt that his legs, especially the knees, were becoming weaker and that he was losing full sensation in his legs. He said, 'It's like I can't quite feel the ground the way I used to.'

Roger hated the winter and loved the summer. This was not surprising, but when I asked him how he protected himself against the cold, he was somewhat puzzled. In one sense he associated the aches and pain with the cold and in another he didn't. He wore what he thought were warm clothes. But if he was working outside and feeling cold, he would finish a job rather than go in the house and get warm. He said that getting the job done was more important. He also knew that he felt less well in damp weather, but he somehow had not connected dampness with the discomfort in his back.

I am stressing Roger's attitude to cold and damp because they were both major causes of his pain. It is as if he knew that, but could not quite accept it. A main part of the diagnosis was 'Wind, Cold and Damp invading the back'. The stiffness, being worse in the morning and feeling worse in damp weather indicated Damp. The contracting pain, and his hating the cold indicated Cold. There was, of course, an underlying deficiency, described as Kidney Yang Deficiency, which made it easier for the Pathogenic Factors to invade.

Roger had several signs of constitutionally weak Kidneys. His face had a bluish/black colour to the sides of his eyes. Even when talking about subjects of interest, such as his daughter or farming, his voice was flat with very few changes in pitch. The Chinese called this a groaning voice and associated it with deficient Kidneys. His habits of work were driven by fear – fear that a crop would fail, fear that the animals would become sick, fear that the government would change the subsidies – in general, that the farm would fail and he would not be able to support his family. His response to fear was to work harder and harder. Fear is the emotion associated with the Kidneys. Roger had two other kidney symptoms. He frequently felt cold in his lower back and he urinated copiously, many times a day.

The principles of treatment for Roger were to tonify and warm the Kidneys and to clear Wind, Damp and Cold from the back. A secondary principle was to nourish the Blood to strengthen his weakened tendons. Roger was also advised to protect himself better and, for example, when he began to get cold outside, retreat to the house, rather than braving it outside, letting the cold penetrate deeper.

Roger was given a prescription which he sent to the herbal dispensary. He received his herbs, but over the first three weeks he took them only four times. He had insisted that he cook them up himself, but because of the pressure of work it just never got done. This was a difficult moment. I could have asked him to try again, but I was not optimistic. Instead I gave Roger two different pills. Together, these were close to, but not exactly the same as, the original prescription.

Roger returned three weeks later somewhat better. He said his legs were stronger and I realised that he had played down the weakness of his legs. The back still ached, but the sharp pains were less. It was November and the weather had been cold so, all in all, there was some progress. I left Roger with the same pills for another three weeks.

Over the next four months Roger took pills regularly and gradually improved. By April his legs were back to full strength and his back was only rarely achy, mainly after damp and wet weather with working several hours in the rain and wet. It was as if Roger could have become really well, but, somehow, there were other things which were more important. Practitioners sometimes find themselves in this bind – where they have higher hopes for the patient than the patient does for himself.

I saw Roger's wife the following November. She said he was still much better, but beginning to get a bit achy. 'He should really be back on the pills,' she said. 'And', I thought, 'taking better care of himself.'

Elisabeth

Elisabeth came for insomnia. It took a while before she explained about the broken heart. She was 35 and eight years before, her husband of three years left her for his 21-year-old secretary. For him it was a clean break; for her it was a confusing, painful disaster. She did not sleep for months and, for a while, this seemed normal. But the inability to sleep just went on and eight years later she was taking an hour or more to get to sleep and then rarely sleeping more than two to three hours a night. Upsetting dreams would wake her and she would be hot and perspire. After waking she listened to the radio or simply tossed and turned.

She had tried sleeping pills. Several did not work. The ones that did seemed to make her feel less well in other ways. She had restricted herself to 'knocking myself out', as she put it, one or two nights a week.

Sleep deprivation is one of the most important factors accounting for poor physical and mental performance. For most of us, it would be hard to imagine sleeping only two to three hours per night. Elisabeth was used to it. She had continued her job as a secretary, but otherwise withdrew from life. The house was sold and she returned to live with her parents and was still with them. She had taken a variety of tranquillisers and anti-depressants, but none of them made a difference. A brief spell of counselling had made no difference. She plodded on, desperately tired, her body depleted and her mind obsessively returning to her husband's betrayal.

The upsetting dreams, feeling hot and perspiring had come on more in the last two years. She now had a glass of water by the bed and a change of night clothes in case she woke wet with perspiration.

Elisabeth's main pattern was Heart Blood Deficiency. Her Heart was the core of the issue. When first married, she already had some signs of Blood Deficiency, but the shock had made a slight disharmony many times worse.

Aside from the insomnia, Elisabeth had all the signs and symptoms of Heart Blood Deficiency: a pale dull face, poor memory, absent-mindedness, being easily startled, a choppy pulse and a pale and dry tongue.

The herbs for Elisabeth mainly nourished Blood and calmed the Shen. Her progress was good at first and then levelled off. After six weeks, she would sleep through two nights a week. The rest of the week she would get five to six hours. The dreams were gone, but often her sleep was light and it often took more than an hour to go off.

This kind of progress, when symptoms are severe, is often typical. People progress well and then plateau for a period of time. There is still a long way to go. At this point, practitioners have different options. They will invariably question whether the herbs need to be modified. They will often do a small re-diagnosis, just to be sure.

Another option is simply to persist on the basis that the body and mind need time to adjust. In Elisabeth's case this seemed to be true. In Chinese medicine, the capacity for relating to others depends a lot on the Heart. For someone who had enjoyed relationships and loved socialising, she had cut herself off. It seemed wilful, but Chinese medicine would see it more as the response of a weakened Heart. She had often said at the beginning of treatment, 'I just cannot see people.'

However, as the Heart grows stronger, it often takes time to believe that relating is all right again. Testing the strength of your Heart is different from testing the strength of your legs.

Elisabeth persisted. After four months, she went off to sleep in less than 30 minutes and usually slept through the night. More importantly, she had begun to develop a social life with several old friends and had been out to dinner with a man from work. Her Heart and Blood were mending.

Elisabeth took herbs for over two years. She had several breaks during that time. Breaks are often recommended for the progress to settle down. She continued to change and finally resumed a normal life. When I last saw her she was carefully entering a new relationship.

James

James was 19, living at home and studying design at a college of further education. He was a good-looking boy, obviously a body builder, and wearing lots of gold. His mother made his appointment and he gave the impression of being mid-way between a boy living at home and a man ready to enter the world.

His complaint was serious. For four years he had had Crohn's disease and it was gradually getting worse. He was on steroid drugs, and surgically removing part of his intestines had been discussed.

Crohn's is a younger person's disease. Part of the intestines becomes inflamed, often bleeds and ultimately leads to a thickening of the intestinal wall and a narrowing of the passage. There is painful cramping, diarrhoea and often mucus and blood in the stools. Western medicine believes that nervous tension and emotional conflict are often the source.

For James, the cramping and diarrhoea with mucus and blood came in bouts of five to six weeks. As soon as it started, he would take a sufficiently high dose of steroids to stop the bleeding, but it would then take up to six weeks to gradually come off the steroids. Over time he had required higher doses of steroids and had shorter remission times.

The diagnosis of the Crohn's symptoms was 'Damp and Heat in the Intestines'. The underlying weakness concerned the Heart and Spleen.

The Damp and Heat needed to be cleared first. But the weakness of the Heart and Spleen needed to be addressed as soon as possible so that James would be able to deal with the issues of growing up without retaining the tension and resulting Heat in his body. I learned later on that both James's father and the crowd he hung out with were less than tolerant of someone with his sensitivity.

James had just started steroids when he first came. The diarrhoea had just come under control and there is always a clinical judgement to be made about how to combine the herbs with existing drugs. He was given herbs to clear the Damp and Heat and he attempted to come off the steroids, with the doctor's agreement, more quickly than usual. He did so, but this may or may not have been significant.

He was then given herbs to strengthen the Heart and Spleen. The gap before the next bout was much longer and it began in a milder form with no bleeding. The problem was more like this when it first began. So James was given a modified form of the original herbs – less to clear Heat and more to strengthen the Spleen and stop diarrhoea. This time he avoided going on steroids and we both agreed that treatment was getting somewhere.

Progress after this was good, but James still moved between good times and times where his bowels were loose and seemed to be heading towards the old pattern of blood, mucus and steroids. Over 18 months he only required the steroids once. He kept several bags of the herbs to clear Damp and Heat in the intestines at home, just in case.

James first came three years ago. I now see him once every three or four months. He has learned a lot about himself and his sensitivity, not least of which is to appreciate who he is and not feel shamed by the expectations of his friends or his father.

People sometimes ask in a case like this what the strengthening herbs do. My belief is that they strengthen an Organ or a Substance and in so doing they make the patient able to function normally. 'Normally' here means being able to learn and adjust and adapt to themselves and to the world, just like most of us are doing a lot of the time. But without that return to 'normal', a person remains overwhelmed, not learning, not adjusting and not adapting, and in James's case suffering inflammation and bleeding. The mental, emotional and physical malfunction all go together. With too much emotional distress adaption declines; distress deepens and the body malfunctions.

We have looked at several patients. It is now time to examine the herbs the patients take.

5

The Herbs and the Formulae

We will now take a look at the individual herbs and the formulae or groups of herbs which the herbalist uses. Chinese herbal medicine is based in the individual herbs, but almost always prescribes a formula or groups of herbs. The reason for this is that the subtle blend of the actions of the individual herbs produces a greater overall healing action.

What is a herb?

The first *materia medica* published after the liberation of China in 1949 was translated as *The Handbook of Traditional Drugs*. In it were listed 475 Substances, which were broken down as follows:

- Fruits: 130

- Roots: 120

- Leaves and stems: 50

- Animal parts: 45

- Flowers: 40

- Minerals: 30

- Stems: 25

- Bark: 20

- Leaves alone: 15

So although we talk of *herbal* medicine, some of the materials used are mineral or animal Substances. These are a small part of the repertoire and, in spite of the potential confusion, we refer to them all as herbs. Of course, they have been chosen because they have a healing action.

Vegetarians may be concerned to hear that animal parts are used. If you are a vegetarian, you should let your herbalist know. Only a few formulae contain animal parts and there are always plant substitutes. Many practitioners in the UK, especially those registered with a professional body (see the Appendix), use no animal parts from endangered species and in practice will use no, or only a few, animal Substances at all.

The general characteristics of herbs

There are some terms which are useful when talking about individual herbs and formulae. Generally speaking, but with some exceptions, most herbs have been *cultivated*, *harvested* and *processed*. The purpose of these processes is to maximise the herb's effect. In addition, they all have properties – *taste*, *temperature*, *direction* and *channel entered* – and they all have *actions*, that is, the effects the herb has on the Organs, Substances and Pathogenic Factors. Often the action is 'explained' by the herb's taste, temperature, direction and the Organ affected. A herb or formula also has *indications* and *symptoms* which are the bodily or mental conditions affected.

We can now look at some of the processes by which herbs are prepared.

The process: cultivation, harvesting and processing

CULTIVATION

Cultivation is the growing of the plant. Some plants are only sought in their natural surroundings. Some are cultivated, which involves considerable knowledge in selecting the seeds, splitting roots, grafting, fertilisation, irrigating and other agricultural approaches. In the lush regions of southern China growing plants for herbal medicine is a major industry.

HARVESTING

When harvesting, different parts of a plant are taken. For example, 'dang gui', or angelica, is a plant known both for 'nourishing' the Blood and 'moving' the Blood. The 'head' or the uppermost part is the 'Blood-nourishing' part, while the 'tail' or the root is the 'Blood-moving' part. In many cases with other plants, only one part is ever used, such as the fruit or the stem.

The time of harvesting often depends upon the part of the plant being collected. For example, roots grow below the ground and are most powerful in late autumn and early spring when they store more nutrients. Barks are collected in February and May when their moisture and nutrient content is highest. Leaves are gathered just before the flowers bloom or in autumn just before they drop. Flowers are picked between March and August when they are in bud or just after blooming. Fruits are picked as they ripen, although a few are picked specifically before they ripen. Seeds are collected after they have matured. This timing is to ensure the potency of the processed herb.

Processing

This comes after the harvesting. The various purposes of processing are to ensure that the final product is clean, easily stored, easily prepared by the herbalist, maximally strong, has side-effects minimised, and has some of its potential clinical effects enhanced.

Processing is said to have three stages. One stage is cleaning and sorting. The next stage is the cutting, pulverising or slicing, often using water to moisten and soften the plant. The third stage uses heat and water, alcohol, vinegar, honey or salt to further process the plant.

For example, 'qing pi' is immature orange fruit. The fruit, which is small, is picked in July or August before it is ripe. It is then cut in half and dried in the sun. It is then soaked in water overnight, cut into slices and again dried in the sun. 'Fu zi', which is the root of the aconite plant, is dug up in July and August and prepared with salt to alter its otherwise toxic effects. Roots are normally dried in the sun or indoors by a fire. Aromatic herbs such as mint are dried in the shade so as not to overdry and lose valuable properties. Animal parts are steamed to kill parasites and bacteria before drying. Each Substance is processed differently.

It is amazing, without the aid of modern chemistry, that the processors learned how to change the actions of a Substance. Chinese foxglove plant is an example. The root is gently heated on hot bricks until the centre is dry. It is then cut into slices and further dried in the sun. This is called fresh rehmannia and has strong cooling properties and is said to clear Heat. To create 'prepared rehmannia', the dried rehmannia is then soaked in rice wine and steamed until it is black. The black indicates the decomposition of a component called catapol. The steamed root, which is black and moist, is a strong tonic and nourishes the Yin.

The properties: taste, temperature and direction

TASTE

Tastes are classified as pungent, sour, bitter, sweet or salty. 'Pungent' is also called 'acrid'. The taste can be neutral and is called bland. The following table gives the taste, the effect of the taste in the body, and a typical food which has that taste.

Taste	Function of taste	Herbs or foods with this taste
Pungent	Disperses, invigorates, promotes circulation, accelerating	Cinnamon, cayenne, ginger, mint, pepper, onion
Sour	Absorbs, consolidates, astringes, hold in, contracts	Crab apple, gooseberry, lemon, lime, vinegar
Bitter	Disperses, eliminates, descends, dries	Coffee, pumpkin seeds, rhubarb, watercress, Angostura bitters
Sweet	Tonifies, harmonises, moderates, expands, relaxes	Bamboo shoots, potatoes, corn, rice, beef, chicken, eggs, liquorice, molasses, soya milk
Salty	Densifies, concentrates, breaks up lumps	Salt, seaweed

The above connections between taste and function do not hold in all cases, but nevertheless have guided many herbalists in originally assessing the potential effect of the herb. Cinnamon and ginger are pungent and you might imagine the effect of these to disperse and invigorate the energy. Cinnamon, for example, is used to disperse. A common cold is described by the Chinese as an 'invasion of

Wind and Cold'. Cinnamon disperses the Wind and Cold and thereby affects the cold.

The sour taste makes your lips pucker or tighten up. This feeling is also the effect of many of the sour herbs – they are said to hold things in that previously were leaking out. Thus, they are used, when appropriate, for a variety of 'leaking' symptoms such as diarrhoea, vaginal discharge, and urgent and frequent urination.

Watercress and Angostura bitters are probably the most familiar bitter tastes. The root of rhubarb is bitter and is used primarily for constipation, to eliminate and to descend.

The sweet herbs are mainly ones which tonify. The greatest tonifier of all, ginseng, is classified as sweet. For most of us who were raised on white sugar, the sweetness of ginseng or corn or chicken or soya milk is not so obvious. To a cultivated palate, however, these would all be considered sweet.

The salty taste is that of table salt. Again, our palates have been spoiled by having so much of such a pure taste, that the herbs that are said to be salty might not be recognised as such by most of us. Many of the herbs which soften lumps that form in the neck are said to be salty.

TEMPERATURE

The gradations of temperature are from hot to warm to neutral to cool to cold. These do not refer to the actual temperature of a Substance, as taken by a thermometer, but the effect it will have on the body. For example, certain curries are known to be hot and they easily increase the heat of the body and make a person sweat. Other foods, such as cucumber, melon, yogurt or cottage cheese are cool. Many people who are Yang Deficient, or short on the warming type of energy, may eat cold foods and have great difficulty digesting them. They really need warmer foods which will warm up the digestive system rather than cool it down. The effect of warming Substances is generally to increase the heat of the body; the effect of cold Substances is to reduce heat, for example, in the case of a fever or infection.

DIRECTION

Traditionally, Substances have also been classified by their direction: ascending, descending, floating and sinking. These again were determined by the taster and then tested out in practice.

Substances with floating or ascending properties make the energy go upward and outward. They might be used to cause vomiting or sweating in order to create beneficial effects. Substances that descend and sink conduct the Qi downward and may bring heat down from the head and calm the mind or promote urination or a bowel movement. Flowers and leaves that are light in quality tend to float or ascend. Seeds, fruits and minerals tend to sink or descend.

Primary actions: strengthening and clearing

A herb may have several actions, but its main one is usually either strengthening or clearing. What is strengthened is the Substances or Organs as in the actions: 'nourish Blood' or 'tonify the Spleen'. What is cleared or got rid of is the Pathogenic Factors as in the actions 'clear Damp', 'resolve Phlegm' or 'clear Heat'.

This two-pronged approach, clearing and strengthening, is one of the great strengths of Chinese herbal medicine. We will look first at three herbs that strengthen and then three that clear. These are simply examples, chosen from literally hundreds of possibilities.

Strengthening herbs

Strengthening herbs mainly tonify Qi and Blood. Although food provides day by day energy, herbs strengthen us by improving the Organs which are the factories that produce the Qi and Blood. Each section on a herb will begin with a short summary of the basic information about the herb.

GINSENG

Common name	Ginseng
Chinese name	Ren shen
Botanical name	Panax Ginseng
Where grown	China, Korea and America
Part(s) used	Root
Harvesting	Dug in the autumn after 6–7 years' growth
Preparation	Cleaned, dried in sun, steamed or baked, cut into slices
Taste	Sweet
Temperature	Slightly warm
Organs affected	Lungs, Spleen, Kidney

Ginseng is probably the most revered strengthening herb. In *The Divine Husbandman's Classic* referred to in Chapter 1 and first published 2000 years ago, it was said:

> Ginseng is a tonic to the five Organs, quieting the animal spirits, stabilising the soul, preventing fear, expelling the vicious energies, brightening the eye and improving vision, opening up the heart, benefiting the understanding, and if taken for some time will invigorate the body and prolong life.

That sounds impressive, if not specific. What the *materia medicas* of today say is that ginseng strengthens the energy of the Kidneys, Lungs, Heart and Spleen. This means that the following kinds of symptoms will be affected: basic tiredness; urinary frequency and urgency; weakness of the legs; deafness; tinnitus; impotence; infertility; heaviness and a 'couldn't care less' attitude; erratic or poor appetite; loose bowels; weak breathing; easily getting short of breath; weak voice; easily catching colds; daytime sweating without physical effort; palpitations with anxiety; insomnia; forgetfulness; restlessness.

The belief that ginseng is to be revered is based on its effect in relieving these kinds of symptoms over almost 2000 years. An American author writing on ginseng said that it 'possesses "non-specific" restorative qualities which strengthen the stress mechanism...and increases its efficiency'.

Research bears this out. Ginseng has been given to mice in controlled studies and it has been shown that: 1) it prevented weight changes in the adrenal, thymus, spleen and thyroid of mice that had been stressed, and 2) it raised the ability of mice and rats to adapt to exceptional stimuli (high and low temperatures) and to accelerate the return to normality from the changes created by various stressors. This is probably the physiologist's equivalent of 'non-specific restorative qualities'.

Ginseng also has a popular reputation as promoting sexual vigour. Research has indicated that there may be some basis for this claim. Ginseng contains saponins which have been shown in recent studies at McMaster University, in Ontario, Canada, to dilate the blood vessels. Poor blood supply to the penis and pelvis is thought to be the cause of both impotence and a lack of arousal. So saponins may explain ginseng's reputation as a sexual tonic.

What is the plant like? There are several varieties of ginseng grown, but we are referring now to the Chinese type. This plant is a smooth perennial which grows about two feet tall. A single stalk rises up from the root and turns into a single leaf which divides into several fronds which in turn divide into small leaves. At the top is a cluster of yellow-green flowers with red berry-like fruits. The plant is cultivated from seed and grown under a bamboo shade. When growing, the flowers of the plant are pinched back to send energy back to the root. The root, the valuable part, is harvested from plants at least five years old.

CHINESE ANGELICA ROOT

Common name	Chinese angelica root
Chinese name	Dang gui
Botanical name	Radix Angelicae Sinensis
Where grown	China, best from Gansu province
Part(s) used	Mainly root
Harvesting	Dug in autumn after several years' growth
Preparation	Root cleaned, smoked and cut into slices
Taste	Mainly sweet, slightly pungent
Temperature	Warm
Organs affected	Heart, Liver, Spleen

Chinese angelica root was first recorded in the original *Divine Husbandman's Classic*. It has appeared again and again in later *materia medicas* and today, is one of the most used Chinese herbs. It has also been used in the West, by European herbalists and Cherokee medicine doctors.

There is a folk tale about its origin. A young couple married, but soon after the husband was required to go off into the mountains to prove himself. The couple agreed that if he did not return in three years, she should remarry. He failed to return and she remarried and shortly after he did return. They were both heartbroken and the wife became sick and weak. The former husband gave her a root which he had brought from the mountain and she became well again. The people of the village called the root 'dang gui' which meant 'should come back' or 'the proper order of things'. The 'proper order of things' is understood today as Qi and Blood in their proper balance – returned to harmony by Chinese angelica root.

The action of the root is to 'nourish Blood' and also to 'move the Blood'. So it is used when there is a Blood Deficiency and when the Blood is stuck and creating pain. It is therefore used a lot for abnormal menstruation, especially where women experience pain (from Blood Stagnation), scanty or no blood flow, continuous uterine bleeding, dull headaches after the period, dizziness upon standing and muscle cramps. You may remember from Chapter 3 that women tend to develop Blood Deficiency more than men. So frequently, angelica root has been thought of as a women's herb. The herb is also said to 'moisten the Intestines' so it deals with constipation caused by dryness.

Europeans have used the root for menstrual problems and, curiously, for flavouring the liqueurs Benedictine and Chartreuse. Cherokee Indians used it for menstrual pain and for 'nervous and weak females' which undoubtedly referred to the Shen Disturbance from a Blood Deficiency.

The growing and processing of angelica root is a slow and painstaking process. It grows best in a cool, moist environment with deep sandy soil, high in organic materials. It frequently takes more than four years before harvesting. It is started from seed and in the first winter the seedlings are taken out of the ground, kept in a cool, dry place, and then replanted in the spring. As with ginseng, the flower buds are pinched back in order to return more of the plant's energy to the root. When the plant is three to four feet tall, the thickened, branched root which is four to ten inches long is taken out of the ground. The root is cleaned and hung from the ceiling and dried first with a smoky fire which gives the root a yellowish-brown colour and then with an ordinary fire until it is 70 to 80 per cent dry. It is then sliced.

Chinese angelica root was used in the prescription for Carol, the lady in Chapter 4 who had severe period pains.

CHINESE DATES

Common name	Chinese date, or jujube
Chinese name	Da zao
Pharmaceutical name	Fructus Zizyphi Jujube
Where grown	China, various provinces
Part(s) used	Fruit
Harvesting	Autumn when fruit ripens
Preparation	Baking or drying in the sun
Taste	Sweet
Temperature	Neutral
Organs affected	Spleen, Stomach

Chinese dates are somewhat similar to the dates we know in the West. They are eaten in China as Westerners might eat apples and are really an overlap between a herb and a food. They have a long history, however, as a medical herb in that they were mentioned in *The Divine Husbandman's Classic* in the superior category. The date itself is a one-inch long oval fruit and is included in a formula, not measured in grams, like other Substances, but in pieces.

Dates have several actions. The first is a general Qi tonic strengthening the Spleen and the Stomach. As you know by now, the effect of a Qi tonic is to improve tiredness, poor appetite, loose bowels and shortness of breath.

The second action is to nourish Blood and settle the minds of those people who feel dispirited and whose emotional life goes up and down. You will remember from Chapter 3 how the Shen resides in the Blood and the Shen is shorthand for our mind.

The third action is probably the one for which dates are most commonly used. They appear in a great many formulae because they moderate the harsh properties of other herbs. They harmonise the flavours, and therefore actions, of the other herbs.

Research supports the view that dates both strengthen the Qi and moderate the harsh effects of other herbs. Dates have been shown to increase the strength or endurance of mice. One group of mice were fed a preparation of dates for three weeks. These mice and a control group were given a swimming test and the mice eating dates showed significantly greater endurance.

The moderating effects were demonstrated on rats. One half of a group of rats who had been poisoned by carbon tetrachloride were given a date preparation. Compared to the other half, this group recovered significantly faster. These same dates are known to contain vitamins A, B2 and C along with calcium, phosphorous and iron.

Those who are interested in animal rights need to know that many herbalists in the West would not support research that involves animal distress, nor do they advocate the use of animal parts that involves the 'harvesting' of animals. The research is often a Western idea, although the Chinese themselves have never worried about using animal material in their herbal repertoire.

These dates come from a small deciduous tree or large bush which grows up to 30-feet high. The fruit is about one inch long and a brownish red to red colour. The dates are beaten from the trees when the fruit ripens in September and October. The best dates are moist, thick-fleshed and red.

Other parts of the tree have also been used. The seeds of one variety of date is a common herb to 'calm the Spirit' and help people who cannot sleep. The root, leaves and bark are also used, but more in one part of China as folk remedies for a wide range of problems.

These are a few of the strengthening herbs. We can look now at some of those which clear Pathogenic Factors.

Clearing herbs

Herbs that clear get rid of some Pathogenic Factors. In Chinese medicine, the list of Pathogenic Factors is relatively short: Wind, Cold, Heat or Fire, Damp, Phlegm, Stagnation of Qi and Stagnation of Blood. Clearing herbs have an effect on these undesirables. The actions are expressed in different ways but some examples are: 'clear Heat', 'transform Damp', 'resolve Phlegm', 'expel Wind', 'move Qi' (for Stagnation of Qi), 'regulate Blood' or 'move Blood' (for Stagnation of Blood).

Let us look at some specific examples.

SCUTELLARIA

Common name	Skullcap root or scute
Chinese name	Huang qin
Pharmaceutical name	Radix Scutellariae Baicalensis

Where grown	China, various provinces
Part(s) used	Root
Harvesting	Mature root cut spring or autumn
Preparation	Fibrous roots dried in sun
Taste	Bitter
Temperature	Cold
Organs affected	Gallbladder, Large Intestine, Lungs, Stomach

Skullcap or 'scute' is a perennial growing about 15 inches high with blue and violet flowers. The fibrous root is used and has four main actions.

The first action is similar to the kudzu root, to clear Heat and drain Fire. It does this especially in the chest region and so deals with symptoms such as high fever, irritability, thirst, and a cough with thick yellow sputum. The most typical Western problem would be bronchitis or the 'Lung Heat' which sent Peter to bed (see Chapter 4).

The second action is to clear Heat and dry Damp. This implies that there are both Heat and Damp. What does this mean? 'Damp', you may remember from Chapter 3, means that there is an accumulation of Body Fluids and the Heat indicates overactivity and usually inflammation. 'Damp-Heat' is usually some sort of acute or low-grade inflammation and this herb deals particularly with acute and chronic infections in stomach and intestines. In the case histories, James's Crohn's disease involved inflammation in the large intestine, and skullcap was one of the herbs used in the prescription he first took (along with kudzu root) when he had diarrhoea with blood and mucus in the stools.

The third and fourth actions are similar and both depend upon clearing Heat. The third is to clear Heat and stop bleeding. Chinese medicine says one cause of bleeding is when the blood gets hot and therefore 'reckless'. Being reckless, it breaks out of the blood vessels. So clearing Heat can deal with the cause of the bleeding. In the case of James referred to above, one of the first changes he experienced after taking the herbs was that the bleeding associated with bowel movements stopped. This was an example of the effectiveness of skullcap (along with other herbs) in clearing Heat which had led to bleeding.

The fourth action is to clear Heat and calm the foetus. There are times when a foetus is disturbed and miscarriage is a possibility where the cause of the disturbance is Heat in the lower abdomen. Skullcap would be used in such a case.

The last action has an aspect of clearing Heat, but it is expressed by saying that skullcap 'subdues Liver Yang'. Sometimes a Liver malfunction is described as a deficiency of Liver Yin energy which results in the Liver Yang (which is warm and powerful) rising up to the head. The symptoms are a throbbing headache, irritability, red eyes, a flushed face and possibly a bitter taste in the mouth. Skullcap would eliminate these symptoms, and it would be used, of course, with herbs that strengthen the Liver Yin energy.

Skullcap grows well in the dry, sandy mountain soils in northeast and southwest China. The best comes from Hubei province and it is only rarely seen in European or American gardens. It is a hardy plant, growing in full sun and easily resisting a drought.

Skullcap is propagated by seed and the roots are harvested in spring or autumn from two- to three-year-old plants. The roots are half dried in the sun and then their bark is scraped off. The roots are then sliced and dried completely.

Skullcap is sometimes further processed by covering the dried slices in rice wine until the root absorbs the alcohol. Later scientific testing showed that the skullcap processed with alcohol retained more baicalin which is thought in

Western scientific terms to be the ingredient which makes skullcap work. This is an example of how traditional processing methods are often vindicated by analytic testing.

GYPSUM

Common name	Gypsum
Chinese name	Shi gao
Scientific name	Calcium Sulphate (Ca SO4.2H2O)
Where grown	China (and the rest of the world)
Preparation	Mineral ground into a powder
Taste	Mainly sweet, slightly pungent
Temperature	Very cold
Organs affected	Lungs, Stomach

Gypsum is one of the minerals of the Chinese *materia medica*. What is this mineral? Most of us live in houses with walls that have been covered with plaster or lined with plasterboard. On a building site, plaster which comes as a powder is mixed with water to create a thick mud which is then applied in a thin coat to a brick or block wall. Gypsum is the powder in the plaster bag.

Gypsum is the key Substance in the 'clear Heat – drain Fire' category. It is one of the coldest Substances in the whole *materia medica*. It is both taken internally and applied externally.

Internally it will be used when an infection is said to have gone to the Qi level. What this means is as follows. Suppose someone gets a cold or the flu. The person may experience both chills and feeling hot. If the illness does not clear up, but gets worse, the main signs in Chinese medicine are called the four 'bigs': big fever, big thirst, big sweating and a big pulse – and no more chills. The big pulse is when the pulse feels strong and is rapid (for example, when the patient is resting), over 90 beats per minute. This often results in a pattern call 'Lung Heat' which Peter in Chapter 4 had. You may remember that after working through his cold, he finally went to bed feeling very hot, with a high temperature, sweating, thirsty and with a rapid, forceful pulse – the four 'bigs'.

Gypsum was one of the herbs he took. Its purpose, along with the other herbs, was to reduce the fever and counteract the inflammation. Such situations are dangerous. Prolonged high fevers can be damaging. In China, the treatment for meningitis is a prescription called 'White Tiger Decoction'; gypsum is the main ingredient.

Gypsum is also used externally on hot abscesses and burns.

GAMBIR VINE

Common name	Gambir vine, stems and thorns
Chinese name	Gou teng
Pharmaceutical name	Ramulus cum Uncis Uncariae
Where grown	China, various provinces
Part(s) used	Stems and thorns
Harvesting	Spring or autumn
Preparation	Dried in the sun
Taste	Sweet
Temperature	Cool
Organs affected	Heart, Liver

This vine grows in China and does, according to our Western ideas, a rather unusual job.

Its first action is to extinguish Wind and alleviate spasms. The Wind we are talking of here is internal, not external Wind. Internal Wind arises from a Blood Deficiency, high temperature or a deficiency of Liver and Kidneys where the Liver Yang energy has risen upwards. It manifests in varying degrees as shaking, twitching, tremors, convulsions, and seizures – in general, uncontrolled movement which often involves muscular spasms. Examples are a simple hand tremor, the shakes of a patient with Parkinson's or an epileptic seizure. These are all internal Wind and this herb is used in each case.

The second action is to drain Liver Heat and subdue Liver Yang. This is similar to the first, but concentrates more on the symptoms which occur when the Liver Yang energy rises: such things as one-sided, throbbing headaches, irritability; red eyes; dizziness; blurred vision; and the frequently associated high blood pressure.

The third action is to release the Exterior. This deals with the type of common cold which is manifesting with more heat than chills and probably a sore throat and red eyes as well. This is called an invasion of Wind-Heat. It is believed that both Wind and Heat are stuck at the level of the protective or Wei level energy. In body terms this is the level of the muscles right under the skin. The stuck energy produces Stagnation which in turn produces Heat. What a 'Release the Exterior' herb does is open the pores and allow the Wind and Heat out. Not surprisingly, sweating often is part of this release. Many other Substances are used more frequently for releasing the Exterior, so the extinguishing Wind properties of gou teng are more important.

Again, research has borne out the views of ancient herbalist. Wind tends to be associated with jerky movements and spasms, where the muscles are tense and out of control. Mice who had a decoction of gou teng injected were found to have many reflexes inhibited. The same decoction lowered the blood pressure of dogs and rabbits. Two decoctions were used, one including and the other excluding thorns. The one which included no thorns was found not to have this effect, bearing out the traditional view that the more thorns, the more powerful the effect. In another experiment, an injection of an alcohol extract of gou teng was found to suppress experimentally induced epileptic seizures in guinea pigs.

The vines are cut in spring or autumn and dried in the sun. Those with more thorns have always been judged superior and are more sought after.

We have now sampled both strengthening and clearing herbs. These herbs are used in formulae and these are our next subject.

Formulae

Formulae are the long established groups of herbs which affect one or more 'patterns of disharmony'. They are not simply several herbs which do the same thing and are added together. They are complex recipes where each ingredient affects the actions of the others. This interaction has been studied for thousands of years and is truly what makes Chinese herbal medicine unique.

As with the herbs, we will look at both strengthening and clearing formulae. We begin, however, by looking at the principles upon which herbs are combined.

Combining herbs into formulae

The question arises: what are the principles for combining herbs together? Imagine you are a cook, about to create a soup which must be both delicious and nutritious. The herbalist is somewhat similar; she is trying to create a formula which deals with several patterns of disharmony. Fortunately, by the time *The Divine Husbandman's Classic* was published (100 BC), guidelines for combining two herbs were already established. Five principles had been established at that time.

FIVE PRINCIPLES FOR COMBINING TWO HERBS

1. Principle one was combining two herbs which have the same effect in order to make this effect stronger. You may remember that 'shi gao' or gypsum is used to clear Heat, for example, when an infection has gone deeper and the temperature is high. In this context, gypsum is used with another herb called 'zhi mu'. The root of this plant also clears Heat so the overall clinical effect is accentuated. The principle is called 'mutual accentuation'.

2. Principle two depends upon patterns of disharmony which naturally occur together. For example, a Spleen Qi Deficiency where the body fluids are not being moved and transformed, naturally leads to the accumulation of Damp. So the weak Spleen and the accumulation of Damp is a naturally occurring double pattern. Two herbs, 'huang qi' and 'fu ling', are frequently used together for oedema, which occurs because of a weak Spleen and an accumulation of Damp. One predominantly strengthens the Qi, the other clears Damp. There are many such patterns which naturally occur together, and the principle here is called 'mutual enhancement'.

3. Principle three is called 'mutual fear'. This is where one Substance, although effective, is also slightly

toxic. The second Substance is used to counteract the first's toxicity. 'Ban xia' or 'pinellia ternatae' is a root which very effectively clears Phlegm, such as the mucus or Phlegm which can accumulate in the nose, throat or lungs. It is, however, slightly toxic and this toxicity is severely reduced when it is used with the fresh root of ginger. Hence, their frequent combined use in formulas.

4. Principle four is called 'mutual antagonism'. This means that each Substance reduces the other's positive effect. In this case, the two herbs are not used together.

5. Principle five also leads to herbs not being used together, and is called 'mutual incompatibility'. This means that used together these herbs create toxicity. In the *materia medicas* where herbs and their actions are listed, there is usually a section called 'Cautions and Contraindications'. This section says if the herb has been found to be 'incompatible' with any others. Naturally these do not occur in formulae.

These principles governed the process of putting two herbs together. In formulae, however, we have six to twelve Substances. So are there rules of thumb for combining the several Substances which go to make up a formula?

Combining several herbs

As well as principles for combining two herbs, the Chinese developed an overall model for how to combine several herbs. The first record we have of this was in the *Nei Jing* referred to in Chapter 1, so these were developed before the birth of Christ. The herbalist starts with a diagnosis and therefore the patterns of disharmony she wishes to address.

So she starts with treatment principles like 'strengthen the Qi and clear Damp' or 'nourish the Blood and calm the Shen'. Suppose she were starting with 'strengthen Spleen Qi and clear Damp'.

The Chinese model was based on the court of the emperor. The first herb will be the chief or 'emperor' herb. This Substance will have a strong effect on the main treatment principle. If this is 'Strengthen the Spleen' we might choose ginseng which was mentioned earlier.

Another Substance will be the emperor's 'deputy'. A deputy will either have the same action as the emperor or it may also have an action against a frequently coexisting pattern. For the deputy in our soup we might choose a herb called 'bai zhu' or white atractylodes. This herb both tonifies Qi and helps clear Damp, thus satisfying both of the deputy's potential jobs.

Another Substance will be called the 'assistant'. An assistant, not unlike an executive's personal assistant, can do several things. It might do the same as the emperor; it might moderate the toxicity of the emperor or deputy; it might, in a complex case, do something necessary but quite different. In this case we will add a herb called 'poria' or 'fu ling'. This herb primarily clears Damp, but secondarily strengthens the Spleen.

Finally, another Substance is called the 'envoy' or 'messenger' or 'guide'. This herb can help focus the overall action of the formula on one part of the body or it can harmonise and integrate the other Substances. Earlier in this chapter we discussed the Chinese date, 'da zao', which harmonises the herbs used with it and moderates any harshness. This would be a good choice, but we will choose instead, Chinese liquorice root, called 'gan cao'. One reason for choosing liquorice root is that it is a good moderator and, as a messenger, it sends the effect of the formula to all Organs of the body.

So we have made a recipe for a soup to strengthen the Spleen and clear Damp. The choice now is quantities. If the Substance is acting as an emperor, it would tend to be used in a larger quantity; if it is an assistant, it would be used in a smaller quantity. We will not deal in detail with actual quantities here except to say that the quantity of one herb in relation to the others can affect its role.

In selecting the above herbs, you may not be surprised to find that you have created a traditional formula, first written down around 1000 AD. This formula is called 'The Four Gentlemen'. The name reflects a habit in traditional Chinese culture which was to refer to four important things that were in harmony and not given to extremes as 'four gentlemen' or 'four noblemen'. A gentleman, from the time of Confucius, is one who exhibits ideal behaviour.

The Four Gentlemen

Ren shen

Bai zhu

Fu ling

Gan cao

This formula is the basic one to tonify Qi. It has many modifications, which have become fully fledged formulae in their own right. For example, although we started out to satisfy the 'clear Damp' principle as well as the 'strengthen Spleen' one, 'The Four Gentlemen' is more for strengthening Qi than clearing Damp.

There is, however, an extension of 'The Four Gentlemen' which does clear Damp. Not surprisingly, it is called 'The Six Gentlemen' and has two more herbs. One of these is 'ban xia' which dries Damp and transforms Phlegm, and the other is 'chen pi' which moves the Qi in the abdomen downwards. Chen pi is the dried peel of orange or tangerine. When Damp collects in the stomach area, it is said that the Qi gets stuck. People will often feel after a big meal that the food gets stuck in their stomach. So a herb which moves the Qi downward is a natural addition.

It is probably obvious that by adding two herbs which move and clear, the resulting formula is, on balance, more clearing than the previous one. Indeed, to 'The Six Gentlemen' we can add more clearing herbs and the resulting formula becomes even more clearing and less tonifying. What should govern this balance?

The patient's diagnosis is the ruling guide. The formula used should match the treatment principles as they apply to the individual patient.

We can now look at a few more strengthening formulae and then some clearing one. The same distinction between strengthening and clearing that we made with individual herbs is the same with formulae. The only difference is that a group of herbs is more flexible and is often created to do a mixture of jobs, both strengthening and clearing.

Strengthening formulae

Strengthening formulae fortify a Substance, such as Qi or Blood or Jing. The actions are: 'tonify Qi', 'nourish Blood', or 'replenish the Jing'. Some formulae act to 'nourish Yin' or 'warm and tonify Kidney Yang' and these are also strengtheners. Many of these formulae will also make reference to an Organ. There are, for example, formulae which 'tonify Spleen and Stomach Qi' and ones which 'tonify Lung Qi'. What they have in common is that they strengthen and thus they include many of the Substances which were labelled 'superior' in *The Divine Husbandman's Classic*.

TONIFY QI

'The Four Gentlemen' and 'The Six Gentlemen', mentioned above, are two examples of 'tonify Qi' formulae. The latter is a development of the former and deals with a greater deficiency which has led to the accumulation of Damp.

The formulae are frequently used with the addition of more herbs to deal with more severe conditions. It is hard to know when to say that you are using a basic formula with a few additional herbs or a new formula which includes the basic one in it.

If we go one step further and add two herbs to 'The Six Gentlemen', we get a formula that does more clearing. The two herbs are 'sha ren' and 'mu xiang'. The former clears Damp from the digestive system and the latter clears the Stagnation of Qi, especially in the digestive system. This one is called 'The Eight Gentlemen' and deals with someone whose Qi is deficient but who also has such symptoms as a feeling of fullness and distension after eating, nausea, vomiting, bringing up sour fluids, loss of appetite or diarrhoea. The Damp is obstructing digestion and needs to be transformed.

STRENGTHENING THE BLOOD

Blood Deficiency comes from three main sources: poor diet; stress, anxiety and worry; and blood loss. Two common causes of blood loss are giving birth and heavy menstrual bleeding. A herbalist will want to understand the reason for the Blood Deficiency as it may well affect her selection of the right formula.

The basic 'tonify Blood' formula is called 'The Four Things'. Again the name is meant to indicate respect for the four ingredients, but, as we lack the same cultural context, the notion is hard to translate. The formula has four ingredients which, like those of 'The Four Gentlemen', have slightly differing jobs. Angelica root was discussed in the herb chapter and I will use the common names for the other herbs.

ACTIONS OF THE SUBSTANCES IN 'THE FOUR THINGS'

Chinese foxglove root	Nourishes Blood and tonifies the Yin
White peony	Nourishes Blood and tonifies the Yin
Angelica	Nourishes Blood and moves the Blood
Chinese lovage root	Moves the Blood

The emperor herb, which is foxglove root, and the deputy, which is white peony, are both herbs which are rich and relatively thickening. When the Blood is deficient, the Body Fluids are often also deficient and the Blood is already 'thick'. Thus, the two other herbs introduce the Blood-moving aspect to balance the effect of the first two.

'The Four Things' would be used for such things as: light-headedness, particularly when standing up; blurred vision; chronic eye strain; sees 'floaters'; pale dull complexion and pale lips; lustreless and weak nails; muscle cramps; generalised muscle tension; constipation; irregular periods; scanty or no menstrual flow; tongue body pale; pulse thin and wiry or choppy.

Many variations are built on the basic formula. For example, where the menstrual cycle is shortened, possibly with severe pain, and the blood flow is copious, dark and sticky, probably with clots, two blood-moving ingredients may be added. This produces a formula dealing with those symptoms.

Some of the other symptoms dealt with by variations or extensions of 'The Four Things' are: threatened miscarriage, painful periods, premenstrual vomiting and nosebleed, sores that bleed profusely and cause insomnia and irritability, dry eyes, photophobia, bad temper, numbness, muscle twitches and infertility. These other formulae have 'The Four Things' in them and have up to eight or more extra ingredients.

Many mental symptoms are also treated via the Blood. Because the Shen functions are mental and the Shen resides in the Blood, treating the Blood often has a large effect on the mind.

TONIFY KIDNEY YIN AND YANG

Another group of the strengthening formulae tonify the Kidney Yin, Yang and Jing. The Kidneys are given great importance in Chinese medicine for three reasons. They store the Jing or constitutional strength, and they are the source of Yin and Yang energy for all the other Organs. Yin and Yang are sometimes spoken of as Water and Fire, Water being the juice or fluidity of the body and mind and the Fire being their warmth and ability to move. Kidneys underpin fertility and sexuality.

There are many different formulae here and the variations depend upon which aspect of the Kidney is weakened and what symptoms the patient is manifesting. Like the Qi strengthening formulae, there are many cases where one formula over time has developed into others.

The typical Kidney Deficiency symptoms dealt with are some of the following, but the formula used will depend upon the exact symptoms and the pulse and tongue.

- Many mental patterns based in fear, for example withdrawal, suspicion, non-exposure, criticising, excessive preplanning.

- Exhaustion; poor stamina; sleeping a lot; poor immune response.

- Difficulties of conception; decreased sex drive.

- Urinary problems.

- Lower back pain or soreness; ache in bones; weakness of the lower back, hips, knees ankles or feet, or legs generally.

- Tenderness in lower abdomen; puffiness of feet or ankles.

- Mental dullness; early decline in sight, hearing and memory.

- Poor bone development; bones fragile; teeth loosening; premature greying of hair; reduced or erratic sexuality.

If you remember Roger from Chapter 4, you will have noticed that many of his symptoms came from a Kidney weakness. The formula for Roger was one which both strengthened Kidney Yang and cleared Wind, Damp and Cold.

We have sampled some strengthening formulae. We can now turn to formulae which clear.

Clearing formulae

Clearing formulae, like clearing herbs, have the job of getting rid of something that does not belong in the person. In Chapter 3 we called these Pathogenic Factors. They are Wind, Cold, Heat or Fire, Damp, Phlegm, Stagnation of Qi and Stagnation of Blood. They block the flow of Qi and Blood and thereby create ill health. We can look first at the invasion of Wind-Cold, which is one form of the common cold.

CLEARING WIND-COLD

This is the Chinese description of one type of common cold. This is where you feel cold, at times cannot get warm, may feel feverish at the same time, your nose runs, and your head and body ache. The Chinese say that Wind and Cold have got stuck between the skin and muscles.

One formula used here is called Cinnamon Twig Soup; the major ingredient is cinnamon twigs, and it is a 'soup' because traditionally the herbs were put in a saucepan and simmered on the stove to produce a cup of fluid to drink.

Cinnamon Twig Soup

Cinnamon twigs

White peony

Fresh ginger root

Chinese dates

Liquorice

This is a nicely balanced formula which mainly clears the Wind and Cold, but at the same time helps to strengthen. The cinnamon twigs are pungent and therefore disperse and promote circulation, thus releasing the Wind and Cold. The White peony enhances the underlying Qi while assisting the Protective or Wei Qi to get rid of the Wind and Cold. The ginger root assists the cinnamon to release the Exterior and also warms. The dates and liquorice strengthen the Qi and the liquorice harmonises the actions of the other herbs.

This formula is frequently varied. For example, if the nasal congestion is severe, the headache bad, or the breathing short, other herbs would be added to deal with these symptoms.

In the West, when infected, we frequently take antibiotics. In energetic terms the effect of these, aside from killing bacteria and stopping the infection, is to make a person more Cold and more Damp. So the original cold is stopped, but the Chinese view is that Pathogenic Factors are not properly cleared and the underlying energy, which has been weakened, is not strengthened. Another approach is to take an over-the-counter cold remedy, which might, for example, stop the membrane in the nose from secreting copious mucus. The advantages of expelling the Wind and Cold with herbs and also strengthening the underlying Qi for the next time, will seem obvious to your herbalist. She will also recommend that keep your underlying Qi strong by having a good diet, taking adequate rest and not overworking – and that you protect yourself by keeping warm.

Clearing Phlegm

We usually think of Phlegm as something on our chest that we cough up. The Chinese notion of Phlegm includes this and calls it external Phlegm. But the overall notion of Phlegm is wider and is applied to almost any accumulation of thickened Body Fluids which are now obstructing the free flow of energy. There is a saying which goes 'Phlegm follows the Qi to accumulate, and there is no place it cannot reach.' Hence, the wide variety of symptoms which get attributed to Phlegm.

Some typical Phlegm symptoms are as follows: vertigo, headache and heavy head; greasy skin and secretions; a feeling of tightness in the throat and difficulty swallowing; thick hands with knobbly joints; chronic chest tightness and stuffiness; palpitations, anxiety and mental disturbance; local heat or cold sensations; chronic clearing of throat and coughing up Phlegm; symptoms getting worse on muggy, overcast, or rainy days or with rapid changes of weather;

abdominal masses (malignant or otherwise) or lumps under the skin. Accumulations of Phlegm accelerate the aging process. The term 'Phlegm' covers the accumulation of many different toxic materials.

One of the basic Phlegm clearing prescriptions is called 'Two Old Soup'. Again, this formula is carefully balanced. The main herb is pinellia or 'ban xia' which was added to 'The Four Gentlemen' to create the 'The Six Gentlemen'. Here it is the emperor herb and is used to transform Phlegm and dry Damp. 'Chen pi', or dried tangerine peel, the other herb which was added to 'The Four Gentlemen' to create 'The Six Gentlemen', is also included. This herb 'moves the Qi' and this is necessary because of the blockage created by the Phlegm. These two herbs occur in proportionally larger quantities than they did in 'The Six Gentlemen' because they are now the emperor and deputy. The other herbs in 'Two Old Soup' clear some Damp and strengthen the Spleen. So this is definitely a clearing formula because of its higher proportion of clearing herbs.

On its own, 'Two Old Soup' is used for the coughing up of copious white sputum, a feeling of fullness and stiffness in the chest, palpitations, nausea and vomiting – basically Phlegm lodged in the chest and abdomen. People who have finished a cold, but are left with a phlegmy chest are often cleared by the use of 'Two Old Soup'.

'Two Old Soup' forms the basis for many other formulae where the Phlegm is more specific to another part of the body. Phlegm clearing formulae are an important part of the herbalist's repertoire. Some of the symptoms addressed by these variations were listed above.

CLEARING HEAT OR FIRE

The Divine Husbandman's Classic said, 'Use cold medicines to treat Heat.' Chinese medicine distinguishes different ways in which Heat or Fire can arise and has created different formulae depending on the type and cause. Heat, a bit like Phlegm, can be associated with differing parts of the body and different Organs as well as different causes. In the internal landscape, Heat is more superficial and Fire is deeper.

We will look at one formula now which addresses severe Heat due to the progress of an infection deeper into the body. You may remember in Chapter 4 when Peter started with an ordinary cold, but worked through it and ended up with a high fever, coughing with yellow sputum, sweating, a rapid and full pulse and a red tongue body with a yellow coating. These are the signs of a pattern called 'Lung Heat'.

One appropriate formula is called White Tiger Decoction. There is a story from Chinese mythology in which a white tiger, who is the spirit of the Metal Element, appears in the autumn, the season associated with Metal, to herald the end of summer's heat. The white tiger symbolises the formula's ability to clear Heat from the Lungs.

White Tiger Decoction

Gypsum

Anemarrhena root

Liquorice root

Gypsum was referred to earlier in this chapter. It is the emperor herb in this formula and it is combined with anemarrhena root which is called 'zhi mu'. This herb was mentioned at the beginning of this chapter when we spoke of how two herbs, with a similar effect, are used together to accentuate each other. These two are an example of increasing the formula's ability to clear Heat. Liquorice root, not only harmonises the action of the other herbs, but in this formula its ability to generate fluids to protect the Yin energy is important.

Why, in a case like this, is clearing Heat so important? If the Heat is allowed to continue, in the end, the Yin energy of the patient is injured. Yin energy is the cooling and nourishing energy and is vital as a balance to the Yang. In the case of Peter, his Yin was injured to a degree and he took herbs to strengthen his Lung Yin energy. Had he not, he would have continued with a greater proneness to colds, an ongoing dry cough, various symptoms of dryness and, for certain, less stamina on the football field. Your herbal practitioner will be interested in making sure you are 'recovered and as good as before', not just recovered.

CLEARING DAMP AND HEAT TOGETHER

Damp and Heat often occur together. Sometimes the source is Damp and Heat invading from the outside, but more frequently it arises from the accumulation of Damp which blocks the energy flow and which finally creates Heat. Damp-Heat can occur in a variety of locations, but common to all are low-grade inflammations and fever, a heavy feeling in the limbs, and a tongue coat which is yellow and greasy. James, one of our case histories, was an example of Damp-Heat in the Intestines. In Western terms, James had Crohn's disease which is an inflammation of the intestines which results in several bowel movements a day and, in his case, often with mucus and blood in the stools.

The formula used initially with James, when the symptoms were bad, was Kudzu, Coptis and Scutellaria Decoction.

Kudzu, Coptis and Scutellaria Decoction

Kudzu root

Scutellaria

Coptis

Liquorice root

Kudzu root is a specific for diarrhoea due to Heat or inflammation in the bowel. It also nourishes Body Fluids which is an important action when the Heat has become chronic. Scutellaria, which we discussed earlier in the chapter, clears Heat and dries Damp and, again, is known specifically to affect inflammation in the intestines. Coptis has similar functions to scutellaria. With James's diarrhoea, the bleeding, which was severe, was the key sign of the Heat (as well as a rapid pulse and a red tongue), and the mucus in the stools was the key sign of Damp (as well as a slippery pulse). The liquorice root in this formula harmonises the actions of the other herbs.

This clearing formula, like many clearing ones, is often used for only a short period of time. When the Damp and Heat, for example, are gone, it is harmful to continue clearing. Once the Pathogenic Factors have been expelled, and sometimes while they are being expelled, the herbalist will be supporting the deficiencies which permitted the Pathogenic Factors to occur.

These formulae – strengthening and clearing – are typical of the herbalist's repertoire. One of the remaining questions is what we can do for ourselves.

6

How Can I Help Myself?

It may be reassuring to know that herbs could help you. But you may also be wondering what you can do for yourself.

If you choose to go to a herbalist, he will undoubtedly, where appropriate, suggest what you can do to improve your health. In this case, having understood his suggestions, you should follow them and test them out. If you are not seeing a herbalist then there are still some things you can do to help yourself with regard to diet and activity. I will describe what I think you can do.

There are also some things that you cannot do, which is to prescribe the herbs for yourself, and I will explain why that is so.

Why it is not advisable to prescribe for yourself

It would be natural to wonder if you can prescribe Chinese herbs for yourself or your family. My view is that self-prescribing with Chinese herbs is not advisable. But I think you should hear why. There are several reasons why self-prescribing looks attractive.

In China many people go to the herb shop and buy pills for themselves or their family. The language of Chinese medicine is definitely part of the common language to a great extent. Many people know some common formulae and many people know folk remedies where herbs are used as an extension of cooking and ordinary nutrition. It is part of the culture to know which foods are warming and which are cooling and to use remedies handed down from mother to daughter. At the same time, one of the recognised causes of illness in China is the taking of inappropriate herbs. The most common example of this is men who wish to enhance their sexual energy and take a Kidney Yang tonic when the warming aspect of this tonic further injures their Yin. But if they can do it in China, why not in the West?

Another reason for this question is that ginseng is readily available in health food shops and advertised for its life-enhancing properties. We described it in Chapter 5 as:

> a tonic to the five Organs, quieting the animal spirits, stabilising the soul, preventing fear, expelling the vicious energies, brightening the eye and improving vision, opening up the heart, benefiting the understanding, and if taken for some time will invigorate the body and prolong life.

You may well wonder, 'Shouldn't we all be taking some ginseng?'

Also, other alternative medicines, notably homeopathy, are available with instructions. In many shops, literature and packaging will instruct you to find the right remedy for your complaint. This is not available for serious illnesses and often books will express reservations about the dangers of self-prescribing. But it is recommended, particularly by the manufacturers of the medicines. The same, of course, happens with vitamins and minerals.

The other reason to self-prescribe is that the herbalist's time costs money. Self-prescribing would be cheaper. So why should you not self-prescribe?

Self-prescribing means going from your symptoms, with the help perhaps of a pamphlet or label on a package, to finding the right formula for yourself. On the other hand, what the herbalist does is both pay attention to your symptoms and discover your patterns. He gets the patterns in part from your symptoms, but relies on a more detailed description of your symptoms than you would normally think significant, and, in addition, your pulse, your tongue and various other signs. So self-prescribing leaves out the patterns. Does this matter?

Let us take a common reason why people consult either a doctor or a herbalist: for breathing problems or asthma. Asthma, or chronic breathing problems, is thought in Chinese medicine to have several causes. Some involve a simple deficiency, some involve Pathogenic Factors and fullness, and many involve both deficiency and fullness. Described in simple language, these come down to:

- weak Lung energy

- weak Kidney energy

- repeated colds which in part are due to the patient's weak protective energy

- an accumulation or retention of Phlegm in the Lungs causing wheezing with the Phlegm described as either Hot or Cold, and probably associated with weak Spleen energy

- a Stagnation of the energy of the chest through the Liver not smoothing the flow of Qi, which is associated more with emotional issues.

These patterns or 'causes' can overlap, but chronic breathing problems can come from any one of them. It would be possible but difficult to specify just one formula for each pattern and where there are overlaps – like both a Lung and Kidney weakness and an accumulation of Phlegm –

the numbers of formulae would multiply. The beauty of the herbalist's diagnosis is that it relates specifically to you. Self-diagnosis by the user is not practical.

The question may arise, 'Would there be any harm in making a wrong diagnosis?' The answer is, 'Yes.' Not distinguishing clearly between a fullness or deficiency or Hot Phlegm and Cold Phlegm would result in the selection of herbs that would be detrimental.

Asthma, of course, is only one of the many reasons someone might want herbs. If we take the list of problems helped by Chinese herbs in Chapter 5, the same thinking applies. Describing the problem in symptoms terms is not sufficiently complete to get you the right formulae. For all these, Chinese medicine assumes there are different underlying patterns.

How will the herbalist help me to help myself?

As a generalisation, Western culture has got more and more away from the idea that we need to care for ourselves. Our grandmothers and grandfathers had more 'health rules of thumb' than we do. As technology advances and we become richer in a material sense, we fail to look after ourselves and are willing to get ill and then ask for help rather live well and avoid disease.

When antibiotics were discovered and infections could be stopped, the 'magic bullet' notion was supported. The magic bullet notion is that if medicine can get the correct drug to the right location in a person, then almost any disease can be conquered. The more we know about the behaviour of the cells involved in the damage created by disease, the more likely we can find the drug which will put it right. The result has been massive investment in finding drugs to deal with the diseases which sometimes we have created ourselves. This may make us wonder if the responsibility is in the correct place.

There is currently a reaction against this attitude. As well as responding to the demands being put upon it, Western medicine is becoming more prevention minded. Doctors are questioning whether it is appropriate to treat people who are not helping themselves. This is all to the good.

In this climate, Chinese medicine is particularly relevant. An important ingredient of Chinese medicine has always been an understanding of the causes of a disease and using these for improvement and prevention. Every pattern of disharmony used by the herbalist includes an understanding of what might be causing it. In many cases, not all, there are important lifestyle changes for the patient to make.

The causes are classified in three simple ways. The first is those coming from the environment, which are the Six Evil External Influences; there are certainly some new ones in our modern day, for example, pollutants in the atmosphere.

The second is the internal causes or the emotions which, if not regulated, lead to illness.

The third are matters of lifestyle which are mainly to do with activity (rest, exercise and work) and diet (what, how much and how we eat).

Your herbalist will know your patterns of disharmony and he will also have questioned you about your lifestyle. As a result, there may well be recommendations he can make. These will be individual. They may involve protecting yourself more adequately from difficult climates. They may involve dealing with repetitive and injurious emotional episodes. They may involve modifying your diet and activity and rest patterns.

In the *Nei Jing*, this advice was described as part of the treatment and just as valuable as the herbs. The outcome of treatment is that the patient gets better and learns to look after himself – not that the patient stays on the herbs for a lifetime. That was the basis on which Chinese medicine developed. There were no herb suppliers who had a commercial interest in keeping the Chinese people on lifetime prescriptions.

Let me illustrate the nature of what we have called 'education'. I have already said that asthma has different underlying patterns, all of which can lead to breathing difficulty. Assume for a particular patient that the difficulty is based more in a weak Spleen and the accumulation of Cold Phlegm. Then the primary advice will be about keeping warm, what food to eat and how to eat it. Specifically, the herbalist would recommend:

- the foods to exclude and the foods to include

- the temperature of the foods eaten: whether they are warm or cool by nature and whether they are literally warm or cold

- the regularity and timing of eating

- the conditions during and after eating

- keeping warm.

In addition, because the Spleen is the main weakness and there are external conditions (mainly Damp) and emotional contexts which are injurious to the Spleen, the herbalist would also know whether there were other improvements in lifestyle which the patient could address. The 'education' is based on the diagnosis and applies to the individual.

It may seem odd that keeping warm is a serious recommendation. Do people not know enough to keep warm? My own experience is that there are many Yang Deficient patients who need to keep warm and yet dress inadequately and who, for example, will walk barefoot on a cold kitchen floor and later complain of a sore, achy lower back. It is important, while the herbs are enhancing their own ability to generate warmth, that patients learn to protect themselves better.

Suppose, on the other hand, that the breathing problem is related to the Stagnation of Liver Qi. In this case, the advice would concern different aspects of diet and also the expression of emotion, dealing with stress, constraints and scheduling – again, as it relates to the individual.

As a patient, you may not initially value this 'education'. After all, it suggests that you might be doing things which are contributing to your problem and it may indicate changes you would rather not make. Both merit a little consideration.

Two examples stand out in my mind as to how people receive the possibility of change. One lady, who was suffering from disturbed sleep and abdominal pain, loved to take rich food and alcohol late at night. Her Liver was at the root of her problems and on one level she seemed to know that alcohol and greasy and heating food contributed to her suffering. In fact she had told me as much herself.

However, when I suggested she might change this habit, over several sessions we ended up in a parent and naughty child relationship. I was the parent, she was the naughty child. She would have loved me to find the formula which allowed her to continue her harmful diet.

I changed my approach. I told her that her dietary habits were affecting her, but that personally I thought she should continue to eat the way she wanted, even to increase it a bit if it pleased her, and only when she was completely sick of her pain and disturbed sleep should she make any changes. She was thoroughly angry with me for a short period of time, but rapidly made changes which did affect her progress.

The other case was also to do with diet, but the response was different. A couple were bringing their young child for treatment. After several visits, the father showed me his hands which were cracked and oozing and asked if I could help. He had caught me at a busy moment and I said that maybe on their next visit I would try to find some time for him and prescribe some herbs. I did, however, take his pulses and I suggested that he should not be eating certain foods. His wife began to giggle and say that they were the only foods he liked. I listed them quickly and I noticed her writing them down. I forgot the incident. When the father returned two weeks later he went to shake my hand. I was puzzled as he had never done this before, but took his hand and then remembered the previous visit. His hands were 75 per cent better. He was a delivery man and the problems with his hands were interfering badly with his work. He had simply done what I had said and, even to my surprise, his hands were so much better. This was one minute's advice and many months of improvement.

The first case taught me how important the delivery of the 'education' is. The second taught me not to underestimate the patient's behaviour and overestimate the herbs.

The question pops up, 'How much change do we expect from the herbs and how much from changes of diet, rest, lifestyle and so on?' There is no general answer which applies to all people. Frequently, people need some change from the herbs before they are able to make any other changes. This response is very individual.

What we know for sure is that most people have some benefit to gain from changes only they can make – and some have a lot more. The issue, if you are considering taking herbs, is whether you are willing to take the responsibility which is yours..

The aim of the good herbal practitioner is to make his patients completely independent and self-sufficient. Once the herbs have done their job, independence and self-sufficiency comes from the patient putting the 'education' into practice. Being proactive rather than passive. This means understanding and making the suggested changes. It means learning to read the signs of impending disharmony earlier and earlier, so that remedial action can be taken. And when defensive action has been taken a sufficient number of times, to make strategic changes so that such problems simply do not occur.

So, when you go to a herbalist, expect to learn something more about caring for yourself. What you do with it is yours.

So what can I do without a herbalist?

There are two main areas where many of us in the Western world can easily improve our health. One is diet. The other is our level of activity.

Diet

The best diet for you depends upon knowing your tendency towards one pattern or another. But there are some general purpose rules.

- It is important to eat regularly. Of course, it is all right occasionally to miss meals, but generally the Stomach likes regularity.

- It is best to eat larger amounts earlier in the day and smaller amounts later; as in the old saying, 'Eat like a king at breakfast, a prince at lunch and a pauper in the evening.' It is obviously not a good idea to eat a large, heavy meal late in the evening when the Organs of digestion, the Stomach and the Spleen/ Pancreas, are relatively tired.

- It is important to chew your food well. The digestion process begins in our mouth and chewing helps release enzymes which are important for the breakdown of the food. Western naturopaths have always said to 'drink your food', meaning that you should chew your food enough that it becomes a liquid before swallowing.

- Eat the right amount. Don't undereat or overeat. Undereating means you use your reserves. Over-eating, which is a prevalent Western habit, tends over time to weaken the digestive process and create Damp.

- Eat under relaxing, calm conditions and have time to continue the relaxation after eating. The digestion process is carried out better when we are not diverting our body's energy into some external task.

- Eat clean and fresh food. 'Clean' means free of pesticides, preservatives, chemicals and hormones. 'Fresh' means when it still has vitality. This is becoming a more and more difficult rule to follow.

- In general, and subject to some exceptions, eat warm food and drink warm drinks. Digestion takes place at around 100°F and cold food and drinks take digestive energy simply to warm the food. Regular cold food over time will cause discomfort and pain.

- In general, eat gently cooked food in preference to raw food. Cooking initiates the breakdown of food and, on balance, in spite of the reduction in food values caused by cooking, the digestion of warm, cooked vegetables will result in more nutrition for the person.

- Pay attention to food temperatures. Use a list of the temperatures of food (the temperature they tend to create independently of their actual warmth) to guide the choice of food. (See Further Reading for this kind of information.)

- If we divide food into 1) grains and complex carbohydrates; 2) vegetables and fruits; 3) animal protein and dairy products; and 4) fats, oils and sweets, it is preferable to eat more of the former groups and less of the latter. That is, the bulk of our diet should be grains, beans, vegetables and fruits with small amounts of animal protein and dairy products and even less of fats, oils and sweets.

- Avoid excess stimulants such as coffee and tea, excess alcohol and recreational drugs. Stimulants damage your Yin energy. Alcohol creates Damp and Heat. Recreational drugs, although it is hard to generalise, over time damage the Liver and to a lesser degree the Heart and Kidney.

As these are general rules, you will have to make many judgements to apply them. A useful exercise is use a notebook and write down everything you eat and drink for a week. Then, as if you were dealing with someone else – someone you care about – take out the notebook and the above rules. Work out one or two improvements that you know you can achieve and make them part of your eating pattern. Give it two months and evaluate any changes.

Activity

This refers to your work, exercise, rest and sleep. This is an area where, in the West, many of us tend to have an excess work pattern. This pattern gets built into our lives and gets justified in terms of income, mortgage payments and many other factors. We spend our energy like a credit card user and forget the Chinese notion of Jing and the regular replenishment of our daily energy.

It is not easy to formulate simple rules here simply because not everyone thinks about, for example, work and play in the same way. It would be useful, however, to make the following distinctions. 'Work' for most people is what we do to earn a living or develop self-respect, but it is usually scheduled in and something we 'have to do'. It may be more physical or more mental. 'Relaxation' is pleasurable time doing whatever we enjoy; ideally, in some sense, we should feel renewed by it. 'Exercise' is deliberate movement which is often more physical (on an exercise cycle watching TV) but can be done with body and mind coordinated and can at the same time come under the heading of relaxation. 'Sleep' means time in bed or napping in a chair. Some useful rules are the following.

- Develop a balance of work, relaxation and rest within one 24-hour cycle. Do not, for example, work yourself into the ground for days or weeks and only then take a break.

- Get adequate relaxation each day, that is, time which you enjoy and where you are not under pressure.

- Get sufficient rest each day. This may be achieved by various combinations of napping and sleeping, but if you are tired when you wake after your main rest, consider as a possibility that you are not taking enough rest.

- Get some exercise each day and preferably enjoyable exercise which coordinates your mind and body – as opposed to exercising just your body and allowing your mind to drift. Chinese exercise such as Qi Gong and Tai Ji Quan are both gentle but combine body and mind together; so would various forms of dancing. Ideally, if your work is not balanced between physical and mental, your exercise can help redress the imbalance.

- If physical exercise makes you feel better, but only for a short while, consider that you have some Pathogenic Factor (which the exercise moves) and some Qi Deficiency which needs addressing.

Emotions

It is not the purpose of this book to give emotional help. But it will be useful to understand the Chinese way of looking at emotions. In Chinese medicine one of the recognised causes of disease is emotions. This is not to say that normal emotions will cause disease. There are times to be joyful, times to be angry and times to experience grief, and so on. Moving through an appropriate emotion is simply part of life.

Disease is caused by emotions which are excessive, although appropriate to the context, or excessive and inappropriate to the context. An example of the first would be where someone lives in a threatening situation for some period of time and the resulting habitual fear causes ill health. An example of the second is where, probably as the result of childhood trauma, we frequently experience an emotion and, comparatively speaking, we do so in contexts which are inappropriate. The frequent experience of that emotion affects internal Organs and can cause disease.

This occurrence is described in Chinese medicine in a variety of ways. For example, habitual excess anxiety can weaken the Blood and in turn make the person more Shen disturbed, more liable to greater anxiety and more prone to the other symptoms of Blood Deficiency. Or, habitual excess grief can weaken the Lungs and make the person more prone to grief and more prone to all the other symptoms of Lung Deficiency.

So imbalanced emotions can weaken an Organ and cause disease. What does this mean in terms of helping yourself?

Most people who habitually experience a negative pattern of emotion will not assume this is easy to change. The first step, however, is to acknowledge that these negative emotions are not part of yourself and that they may be limiting or simply debilitating your health. Once you acknowledge this, you will be more motivated to make changes. This can make a big difference.

So one of the first tasks is to review your habitual feelings. If you find habitual negative feelings, simply ask: 1) 'Is it possible that these feelings are affecting my health?' and 2) 'Is it important to me that I continue to have these feelings?' If the answer is that they may be affecting your health, but you do not in fact benefit from them, then start to imagine how well you might be without them. A determination to make changes is a useful starting place.

My suggestion is that you also take advantage of strengthening herbs. There is an emotion associated with all the main Organs. When an Organ is deficient, then the expression of the associated Organ is more likely to be out of balance. For example, joy is the emotion associated with the Heart. When the Heart is deficient, then a person is more like to experience ongoing bouts of sadness. When the Heart is stronger these will recede and the changes we need to make become easier. The better our energy balance, the more our emotions will become normal.

We are nearing the end and need to consider how you might find the right herbalist.

7

How Do I Find a Herbal Practitioner?

If you decide to try Chinese herbs, how do you find a good practitioner? This comes down to research and, once you find one, evaluating what you are getting.

Most patients want both a skilful practitioner and one they feel comfortable with. In this respect, it is useful to listen to the experience of others. Most herbalists live by their reputation. If a friend, or someone else who you trust, describes a good experience with Chinese herbs, then this is a step in the right direction. Ask this person what they went for, how long they took to get better, whether they liked their practitioner, how much it cost and anything else that seems appropriate. Ask whether they would recommend their practitioner or have some reservations.

If the practitioner does not live locally, ask the other person if they could ask their practitioner to recommend one in your area.

After that you might decide to ring the practitioner for a brief chat. This is not always possible. Some practitioners allow their receptionist to make the appointments and do not have conversations with potential patients. In any case, you will be able to ask questions about fees, the costs of the herbs, and how long you should allow for appointments. You can also ask at this stage whether the practitioner belongs to a professional body.

Belonging to a professional body is not a guarantee of excellent treatment, but it does improve the odds. So without a reference, you may approach the relevant professional body and find the name of a local practitioner. In the Appendix I refer to several professional registers. There is not always such an organisation in every country. Being on such a register usually means that the practitioner has a specified standard of education, adheres to an ethical code and follows a code of practice.

When you find a practitioner, there are a few criteria you can use to evaluate how you are treated. The following list outlines these and also tells you roughly what to expect on your first visit. The herbalist should be doing a complete diagnosis. This means that 1) your pulse should be taken; 2) your tongue should be observed; 3) you should be asked detailed questions about your complaint or complaints; 4) you should be asked questions about matters other than your complaint; for example, if your problem is breathing or an emotional issue, you should still be asked about your diet, perspiration, sleep patterns, daily activity and many other similar issues. You may feel that some of these have nothing to do with why you came. A practitioner who never took your pulses or looked at your tongue and did not ask any questions other than about your complaint would probably be working only from symptoms.

One final comment. One of the reasons for finding a practitioner on a professional register is that it is safer. Just as you would want a well-trained surgeon, you want a well-trained herbalist. What are the safety issues?

There are three considerations with the safety of herbs. The first is that the herbs used have been tested over hundreds and sometimes thousands of years. This almost eliminates the worries that accompany modern drugs, which are tested to prove that they will have the desired effect, but cannot be tested exhaustively to eliminate serious side-effects.

The second is a wrong diagnosis and therefore a wrong formula. I said above how self-prescribing in China is a cause of problems because the wrong formula can be chosen. This is also unlikely with a trained herbalist. The traps are well known to practitioners. Training programmes stress the potential problems. For example, if a clearing formula is given, then the trained practitioner will not give an excessive amount but enough to allow the symptoms to be cleared. Otherwise, the patient may be continuing to take herbs which are no longer relevant and may be harmful. There are guidelines built into the Codes of Practice of professional bodies.

The third consideration is where the practitioner makes a correct diagnosis, but prescribes herbs in the wrong quantity. For example, there have recently been cases where Chinese herbs were thought to have caused liver damage. The quantities used were suspected to be in excess of what normal practice recommends. Finding a practitioner who belongs to a professional register ensures good practice. When any such issue arises, the profession takes quick action. Hence, my strong suggestion that you only go to a qualified practitioner.

In the Appendix, I suggest how you might find such a practitioner. Should you choose to do so, I wish you the best of luck in improving your or your family's or friends' health.

PROFESSIONAL REGISTERS

United Kingdom

In the UK there are two main professional registers. The easiest path is to visit the registers' websites where you can find a 'Find-a-Practitioner' section, but you can also telephone and for a small sum receive a list of practitioners.

The website of the Association of Traditional Chinese Medicine and Acupuncture UK is *www.atcm.co.uk*.

The website of the Register of Chinese Herbal Medicine is *www.rchm.co.uk*.

United States

The best contact in the USA is the National Certification Commission for Acupuncture and Oriental Medicine whose website address is *www.nccaom.org*. Although this is mainly an acupuncture website, they have within the site a register of practitioners trained in Chinese herbal medicine.

Australia

In Australia there is one main register of Chinese herbal practitioners, the National Herbalists Association of Australia, which can be reached at *www.nhaa.org.au*. This site also has a 'Find-a-Practitioner' section.

FURTHER READING

The following are some books you might like to consult for further information.

Bensky D., Barolet, R., Ellis, A. and Scheid, V. (2009) *Formulae and Strategies.* Seattle, WA: Eastland Press.

This is a serious textbook covering the formulae used in Chinese medicine. Unless you are a student of Chinese herbal medicine, you are unlikely to read it, but could consult it to find the description of a particular formula.

Bensky, D. and Gamble, A. (1993) *Materia Medica.* Seattle, WA: Eastland Press.

This is a textbook covering the herbs of Chinese medicine. It you want to consult the actions of a specific herb, it would be useful as a reference book.

Hicks, A. (2011) *88 Chinese Medicine Secrets.* Oxford: howtobooks.

Herbal practitioners may well give you diet and lifestyle advice to supplement treatment. This book gives 88 practical ways to improve your health and for that reason is definitely worthwhile.

Hicks, A. (2010) *The Acupuncture Handbook.* London: Piatkus.

This book is an overview of Chinese medicine particularly from the perspective of acupuncture treatment.

Kaptchuk, T. (1994) *Chinese Medicine: The Web That Has No Weaver.* London: Rider.

This is a more extensive introduction to the theory behind Chinese medicine.

Legget, D. (1999) *Recipes for Self-Healing.* Devon: Meridian Press.

This is a practical book on the Chinese principles of diet. It contains theory, recipes and information on selecting the best foods and choosing foods of the right temperature.

INDEX